BODY MASSAGE FOR
THE BEAUTY THERAPIST

By the same author
Care of the Skin

BODY MASSAGE FOR THE BEAUTY THERAPIST

Second Edition

Audrey Githa Goldberg

M. C. S. P., S. R. P.

Formerly Senior Lecturer in Beauty Therapy

Photographs: Sefton Samuels, F. R. P. S.

Illustrations: Jean Perry, A. I. M. B. I.

HEINEMANN PROFESSIONAL PUBLISHING

Heinemann Professional Publishing Ltd
Halley Court, Jordan Hill, Oxford OX2 8EJ

OXFORD   LONDON   MELBOURNE
AUCKLAND   SINGAPORE   IBADAN
NAIROBI   GABORONE   KINGSTON

© Audrey Githa Goldberg 1972, 1989
First published 1972
Reprinted 1976
Reprinted (with revisions) 1979, 1982, 1986
Second edition 1989
Reprinted 1990

British Cataloguing in Publication Data
Goldberg, Audrey Githa
Body massage for the beauty therapist
2nd ed.
1. Beauty care in massage
I. Title

664.7′2

ISBN 0 434 90659 x

Printed in Great Britain by
REDWOOD PRESS LIMITED
Melksham, Wiltshire

Foreword

I consider it to be both a pleasure and a privilege to be given the opportunity of writing the foreword to this outstanding text book.

Few technical publications can have contributed more to the education and training of the student than is offered in the following pages.

The author has cleverly combined her obviously extensive knowledge of physiotherapy with the highly specialized requirements of the beauty therapist, and has presented her work in a manner which the reader should readily comprehend.

The elucidation of a subject where technical knowledge and manual movements are so inter-related is never simple, yet Mrs. Goldberg has succeeded in doing this in a most interesting way.

Students and teachers alike will welcome this book—incidentally the first of its kind—and should gratefully accept it as an original and authentic standard work.

L. SHARRAD

Vice Principal
London College of Fashion and
Clothing Technology

Preface

Manual massage in this supersonic moon age of machinery has almost been superseded by electrical devices. But not quite. For although they can indeed produce quicker results which are far less tiring to the operator, no mechanical substitute has yet been found to replace the sensitivity of touch which exists in a pair of well-trained hands, and which is so essential to convey vital information for the correct application of massage.

It seems superfluous to say that it is a form of treatment providing physical comfort and reassurance which is as old as civilization itself. Yet in the past, massage has been badly neglected, misused, derided, and degraded. The beauty therapy profession is rapidly expanding and with it the demand for massage has grown. Most people enjoy the sensuous luxury of a massage especially when well administered, and it is to the beauty therapist that they are now turning for it with confidence.

This book, covering the City and Guilds of London Institute syllabus on body massage for the Beauty Therapist's Certificate, contains a comprehensive and useful chapter about exercises. It has been written for the student, the teacher, and the beauty therapist who wish to learn, to revise, or to improve their standard of massage simply and clearly without confusion. In this connection it will also be found useful by those following courses run by the National Society of Health and Beauty Therapists, the British Association of Beauty Therapy and Cosmetology Limited affiliated to CIDESCO, and other examining bodies.

The therapist in the book is referred to as 'she', and generally the client also; but of course there are many men today who learns and practise the art of massage and who also require the therapeutic effects it can give.

I am most grateful to Mr. L. Sharrad, Vice Principal at the College of Fashion and Clothing Technology, London, for all his help and advice. Also I would like to extend my thanks to Miss Brenda Savage M.Sc., M.C.S.P., Dip.T.P., of the Physical Treatment Centre, Harrogate, for kindly reading the typescript and advising me on several points.

I am most indebted to Miss Hogson, Professional Consultant at the Chartered Society of Physiotherapy for her valued assistance, and to Miss Willis, of City and Guilds of London Institute.

A. G. G.

Preface to Second Edition

Since its publication in 1972, this book has become the standard work for students of body massage in beauty therapy and has been reprinted, with revisions, on several occasions.

This new edition has been revised by my daughter, Lucy Goldberg IEL ITec, a practising beauty therapist, and I know that it would have given Audrey the greatest pleasure to have had Lucy's co-operation on the book.

Several of the techniques have been revised and updated to cater for most examination syllabuses, especially City and Guilds and CIDESCO, and a section has been added on the important topics of aromatherapy and gyratory massage, both of which have come into prominence since the book first appeared.

IVAN J. GOLDBERG

Contents

page

Foreword   v

Preface   vii

Preface to the Second Edition   viii

List of Plates   xiii

1. A HISTORY OF MASSAGE   1

2. ETHICS, THE BEAUTY THERAPIST, AND THE SALON   9
   Qualities of the beauty therapist—Vital requirements for massage—Business organization

3. MANIPULATIONS AND MASSAGE TECHNIQUE   19
   Four groups of manipulations—Technique of manipulations—Stroking manipulations—Pressure manipulations — Percussion manipulations — Shaking
   manipulations—Summary of effects of massage—
   Psychological effects of massage—General contra-
   indications of massage—Lubricants, oils, powder,
   and massage creams—Hand exercises—Hints for
   practising technique

4. THE PHYSIOLOGICAL EFFECTS OF MASSAGE   44
   Effects on the muscles—Effects on the bones and
   joints—Effects on the circulatory and lymphatic
   system—Effects on the lungs—Effects on the skin—
   Effects on adipose tissue—Effects on the nerves—
   Effects on the abdominal organs—Metabolism and
   beauty

5. ORDER AND METHOD OF WORK   52
    Preparation and procedure—Order and method of
    general massage—Programme for full general body
    massage lasting 60 minutes—Detailed technique of
    body massage—Abdominal massage—Modification
    of treatments—Head and scalp massage—Face mas-
    sage—Modification of treatment for head and face
    —Modifications for stiffness in the joints

6. BONES   88
    Classification—The extremities and girdles of the
    body—Bones of the upper limb—Bones of the
    lower limb (leg)—The vertebral column (back
    bones)

7. JOINTS   III
    Classification—Joints of the upper limb—Joints of
    the lower limb

8. MUSCLES   131
    Kinds of muscular tissue—Characteristics of muscle
    fibres—Muscles of the shoulder—Muscles of the
    upper arm—Muscles of forearm and hand—
    Muscles of buttocks and thigh—Gluteal muscles—
    Quadriceps muscles on front of thigh—Other
    muscles acting on thigh—Adductor muscles on
    medial side of thigh—Hamstring muscles on back
    of thigh—Femoral triangle—Muscles of the lower
    leg—Muscles on sole of the foot—Muscle on dorsum
    of the foot—Muscles on the back of the trunk—
    Muscles of neck and chest—Muscles of the abdo-
    minal wall—Muscles of scalp and facial expression

9. PASSIVE MOVEMENTS   171
    Technique

10. ACTIVE EXERCISES   182
Effects and uses on the systems of the body—
Effects and uses on health and beauty—Some
mechanics of body movement—Some important
points for exercise schemes—Order of a general
scheme of exercises—Muscle work, effects, and uses
of the fundamental positions—Programme of exercises—Explanation, command, and cycle of exercise
—Posture—Exercise, massage, and obesity

11. BREATHING AND RELAXATION   234
Mechanics of respiration—Some important points
—Relaxation

12. ABOUT ELECTRICAL TREATMENTS   248
General dangers—Further general precautions—
Galvanic current—Faradism and sinusoidal currents
—Infra-red and radiant heat radiation—Ultra-violet
light—High frequency—Some conditions for treat-
ments—Care of equipment—Hints on orderliness—
Help the client

13. NEW TECHNIQUES
Aromatherapy—Gyratory massage   271

Index   277

List of Plates

The plates appear between pages 66 and 67

1. Effleurage into the femoral triangle
2. Effleurage into the axillae
3. Effleurage to the back
4. Finger kneading
5. Ironing
6. Wringing
7. Skin rolling
8. Frictions round the knee joint
9. Hacking
10. Clapping
11. Kneading the biceps
12. Wringing the triceps
13. Single handed picking up of the biceps
14. Single handed picking up of the forearm extensor muscles
15. Thumb kneading to the hand
16. Wringing the hypothenar eminence
17. Kneading the quadriceps and the hamstrings
18. Alternate handed kneading above and below the knee joint
19. Wringing the calf muscles
20. Thumb kneading to the anterior tibial muscles
21. Stroking the foot
22. Double handed picking up of the neck
23. Divergent hacking over the scapular muscles
24. Effleurage to the supra-clavicular glands
25. Picking up on the back
26. Transverse clapping

27. Beating the buttocks
28. Alternate method of stroking the neck and chest
29. Kneading of the small intestine
30. Stroking the ascending and transverse colon
31. Kneading the abdominal wall

I. *A History of Massage*

The word 'massage' is thought to be derived either from the Arabic for 'press softly' or from the Greek for 'knead'. Massage is a form of treatment, coupled with exercises, which has been passed down through the centuries for thousands of years.

Records show that in ancient China over five thousand years ago there was a system of massage and exercise in use. Archaeological expeditions in Asia Minor have established that ancient Asiatic women and men used perfumed oils abundantly on their bodies and hair. It is almost certain that most races used massage and exercise in one form or another dating as far back as the prehistoric ages of man. The peoples of ancient civilizations in Persia, Japan, and Egypt practised the art of massage for cosmetic purposes, and found that they also gained therapeutic effects when they rubbed oils and perfumes into the body and skin to beautify it. Creams taken from Egyptian tombs were found to contain camel fat, almond oil, sheep fat, or castor oil mixed with various resins and tannic substances. These were for cosmetic purposes and were massaged into the skin. Anointing was the placing of a lump of fat on the head, which would gradually melt in the heat and cover the hair and body. Clothes would then cling to the body and reveal its shape. Anointing was also the expression used for rubbing oil into the body. Perfumed oils were used in three different ways by the ancient Egyptians: as offerings to their gods, as an enhancement of the body's beauty, making it smell pleasantly, and as the main ingredients for embalming the dead.

A great selection of the pots and vessels in which these oils were kept may be seen in the British Museum. They are so pretty that many designs for today's cosmetic jars are taken from them.

The Cretans in 1700 B.C. were great believers in personal hygiene and aesthetic beauty and they oiled their bodies when they took their daily baths. They believed that fresh air was essential for a beautiful body, and were meticulous about good ventilation producing a cooling system of breezes.

In 1000 B.C. Homer spoke in his Odyssey of beautiful women 'rubbing and anointing war worn heroes' to refresh and revitalize them after battle. He also described the toilet of the Greek goddess Hera in the Iliad: 'and with ambrosia first her lovely skin she purified with oil anointing'. The Greeks favoured gymnastics and believed them to be the basis of a good education. Massage, using the essences of sweet-smelling herbs and olive oil, was applied to the body. The Greek women were shy and plump but enjoyed gymnastics, and in order to acquire a graceful body they learnt dancing. Magnificent muscular physique, the Greek attribute so admired today, was due to the importance they attached so long ago to the use of exercise in building up the body.

The ancient Romans ruled by the Etruscans had quite an advanced system of massage also. Slaves always carried oils around in glass containers slung over their arms in case their masters and mistresses wanted a massage. Exercising, bathing, and sunbathing became quite organized in that order, and, as well as looking better, the Romans began to find considerable benefits both physically and mentally. The schemes of exercises which preceded the baths were carefully graded according to the age and fitness of the individual and even catered for their moods. Running, lifting dumb-bells, playing with balls and hoops were especially popular. Following all these gymnastics, sweating in the baths was recommended. The baths were taken in four stages, not unlike the varying systems followed today. First, there was a period of gradual warming-up sufficient to start sweating in mildly heated waters or steam. This led on to profuse sweating for a long period of time in a much hotter temperature. Then this was followed by the cooling-down process of a bath in tepid water. Finally, for those who were more hardy, plunging into icy cold water concluded the bathing. During all this time the slaves were expected to rub down their masters and mistresses. Together with manual massage, small brushes, not unlike curry-combs, were used. These were made of ivory or bone. Metal such as silver, copper, or iron was used if a more stimulating effect was desired, and if the skin could stand it. Sunbathing in the fresh air followed and completed the bathing routine which has changed little throughout the ages. Today certain rheumatic conditions of joints are treated with silver and gold injections and there are many people who wear copper bands in the belief that rheumatism can be prevented or relieved by doing so. Birch twigs are used by the Finns before bathing, and loofahs, scrubbing brushes, and flannels, have replaced the old idea of the curry-comb. A brisk rub-down with a rough towel after a bath or shower is only a modern idea on the old theme.

From these early beginnings of health and beauty a medical school of thought about massage arose. Around 500 B.C. the Greek historian Herodotus applied exercises and massage in the treatment of disease. Principles about the technique of rubbing began to be formulated. Massage was directed away from the heart, the pressure varied during the treatment, starting off by being gentle at first and then becoming deeper and quicker and petering off again slowly towards the end. Greasy mixtures were used.

In all the large cities in Greece at this time gymnastic centres were set up. Beautiful and splendid buildings were erected where students and philosophers could meet to discuss philosophy and attend lectures, whilst bathing and exercising at the same time. Greek games became very important and it is recorded that the body was rubbed and anointed with oil, fine sand, and powder before and after the games took place. Javelin throwing, wrestling, running, and jumping were great favourites. Many of the beautiful ruins of these gymnasia, built during the Greek civilization, can still be seen today in Greece.

Hippocrates, the father of medicine about 380 B.C., really used massage for the treatment of injuries and disease. He found that it was more beneficial if rubbing was done towards the heart, although the circulatory system was not understood then. It would seem, from his emphasis on pressure application, that Hippocrates had discovered the physiological effects of massage that are accepted today. He stated that 'hard rubbing binds; soft rubbing loosens; much rubbing causes parts to waste; moderate rubbing makes them grow.' His observations were very astute, and he advocated the use of a gentle and smooth rate and rhythm. He also advised women to sing at the tops of their voices to improve their bust line.

Galen (130–200 A.D.), a famous doctor during the Roman era, experimented in physiology and discovered that arteries were filled with blood, and not air as previously believed. He varied the direction of massage according to the reason for its being applied, and also greatly believed in treating injuries and diseases with it. Roman gladiators were oiled and massaged until they were glowing red and supple before commencing battle. Around this time some other terms describing massage were pommelling, squeezing, and pinching. The latter was recommended to be used all over the body to relieve neuralgia: a good counter-irritant, no doubt. Public baths modelled on the Greek style of architecture were by now more commonplace than ever before. People would gather together to exchange gossip and news. Being absolute geniuses with water their baths were quite unique. The Romans left their mark in England during the first century A.D. in towns where waters were considered to contain special minerals and salts of health-giving value. Harrogate, Buxton, Bath, Leamington, Droitwich, Cheltenham, Llandrindod all became spa towns famous for their springs, baths, and waters. Sulphur, magnesium, calcium, and peat of the area were utilized by the Romans in the quest for health and beauty. Many of these waters are still taken today and the towns where the ruins of the Roman baths can still be seen remain favourite and delightful attractions for tourists from all over the world.

Little seems to be recorded about massage or beauty again until the early Middle Ages, when wise women would advise on health and beauty. One Italian woman doctor about 1100 A.D.

advised those ladies preoccupied with slimming and beauty to bathe in the sea and use deodorants which were made of herbs. Her remedy for losing weight was to be frictioned all over with cow dung mixed in medicinal herbs, and then to spend a long period of time sweating heavily in a small room, overpoweringly heated by a wood fire. Hot sand baths near the sea provided an alternative method for producing the same effect as the heated chamber. Today in Italy sand 'graves' are still to be seen near the sea in which people bury themselves up to their necks in the hot sand for the curative and slimming effect attributed to heat and sweating. Peat and mud baths are also still prescribed for rheumatism and are used as beauty treatments. Pine is the most popular essence used today in refreshing hot baths; perhaps this replaces the pungent odour of the cow dung.

During the fifteenth, sixteenth, and seventeenth centuries, Switzerland, France, Italy, Prussia, and England produced several famous physicians and surgeons who began once again to use massage in the treatment of injuries and disease. The old terminology of massage remained but new words such as pressure, kneading, and manipulations were introduced. Opinions about pressure were expressed and an Italian doctor even went so far as to state that the position of the patient should be outstretched lying down. Generally speaking, the patients were placed in most uncomfortable positions.

In the seventeenth century strange recipes for lotions and creams could be found to beautify the face and body beyond all hopes and dreams. One such lotion claimed to remove pox marks. It merely filled in the holes left by smallpox and gave an illusion of smoothness. There were quack doctors and beauty counsellors who lived by their wits, and patented medicines, potions, and creams for massage claiming fantastic results. New Bond Street opened its first beauty salon, where women would go, believing that the creams, oils, and cosmetics which the proprietress applied and sold would work miracles on their faces and bodies. These cosmetics were outrageously expensive and the lady was eventually imprisoned for fraudulent claims. Hand creams were fashionable and ladies went to bed wearing chamois leather gloves which were saturated with cream to keep their hands soft and supple. Beauty care and cosmetics were considered to be only within the reach of high-class society, actresses, or the demi-monde. Perfume was coupled with witchcraft, and laws governing the use of cosmetics were made which sentenced women to imprisonment. Massage for beauty at this time did not rate highly and most practitioners were suspect. Some of the pots which were made at this time for oils, grease, unguents, pomades, and lotions had decorative lids which are still in existence, and are eagerly hunted by 'pot-lid' collectors today.

From the end of the eighteenth century a great revival in massage really began. Many authorities wrote and expounded their theories on the subject. One extremist advocated that massage should be given with great violence, and all had different ideas about the terminology, pressure, rate, rhythm, and medium, such as oil or powder to be used, position of the patient, and the duration of treatment. Some advocated dry hands; one used a metal object covered with leather. Some suggested that four minutes' massage to any one area was sufficient; another stated that up to forty minutes could be given. Trial and error was another means of practising massage, and if it had not suited the patient one day a modification was made the next. The massage field became confused from then on with so many different opinions and descriptions. Peter Henry Ling of Sweden (1776–1839) made the most dramatic contribution to massage and exercise at this time. His influence in the early nineteenth century spread throughout all Europe and America. He was a conscientious and devoted worker, and realized that it was important to acquire a certain knowledge of anatomy and physiology before applying massage and exercises to the body. Of medicine he knew little and only treated those conditions he considered to be normal, emphasizing that all other conditions should be reviewed by the doctor. He founded the Swedish system of massage and exercise, and introduced terms such as effleurage, petrissage, vibration, and friction, as well as rolling, slapping, pinching, and several other descriptions of massage. However, despite the good work and promotion of massage by Henry Ling, it was not until the end of

the nineteenth century that massage began to become favoured
and accepted all over the world as an orthodox method of
treatment. Perhaps this was due to the fact that training was
inadequate and poor, and that those women engaged in massage
were generally of ill repute and opportunists.

Doctor Mezger of Holland (1839–1901) helped to establish
massage finally as a reputable means of treatment by prescribing
it widely and practising it himself. Europe and America recognized
and accepted its importance from then on, leaving England to be
convinced. Beauty parlours in Bond Street, where facial massage
became a speciality, began to flourish and their reputation grew.
It was a rare sight by now to see a face unpainted or unpowdered,
and oils and creams for the body and hands at the end of the
nineteenth century were bought by all.

In 1894 a group of women joined together to form the Society
of Trained Masseuses, in order to try and raise the standard and
reputation of massage in this country. Rules and regulations for
training were made. Examinations were set and the Society
flourished.

In 1900 it became licensed by the Board of Trade and was
called the Incorporated Society of Trained Masseuses. During the
1914–18 War its membership increased enormously. In 1920 it
amalgamated with the Institute of Massage and Remedial
Exercise (Manchester). A Royal Charter was then granted and it
became known as the Chartered Society of Massage and Medical
Gymnastics. The title was again changed in 1943 to the Chartered
Society of Physiotherapy. State Registration came in 1964.

So it can be seen that massage was eventually given the stamp
of respectability by the medical profession and the State in the
treatment of injuries and disease, although it is little used in
hospitals today. Although massage in physiotherapy had reached
a high standard, it seemed as though there was an urgent need to
raise the standard as practised in the beauty field.

In June 1966 City and Guilds of London Institute set up an
Exploratory Committee to look into the possibility of providing
further education and training for girls wishing to study beauty
therapy, and of establishing a nationally recognized course. A

syllabus was drawn up by a working party consisting of people from different beauty organizations, the education world, and the medical profession.

In September 1968 the first full-time courses in beauty therapy were offered in four colleges of further education by the Institute, and in May 1970 the first City and Guilds examination in this field was held.

All that remains is for beauty therapy to become a State-registered profession.

2. Ethics, the Beauty Therapist, and the Salon

Qualities of the Beauty Therapist

The essential qualities of being a beauty therapist do not merely lie in the ability to give a good massage, exercises, or any other treatment. To be successful, a therapist must have a strong belief that whatever she is doing is right. This involves a deep sincere liking and interest in the work she has chosen to do. It requires a high level of tolerance of human failings when dealing so intimately with people in this profession, many of whom return day after day, week after week.

Each client is an individual case for treatment and therefore should be regarded as such, and not subjected to an indifferent attitude by the therapist. Beauty therapy is a personal business and the therapist must have the ability to concentrate on the special requirements necessary for each case in hand to obtain the best possible result for the client's total benefit and well-being. The ability to be kind, comforting, and sympathetic, to be tactful and reassuring, to be cheerful and optimistic without ever promising too much should be present at all times in the therapist's disposition. These inherent qualities are an integral part of the treatment and indeed of any therapy. They are better known as the 'bedside manner'. It is often the bedside manner which effects the cure and instils confidence once again into the client. They are the trademarks of professionalism and will help to build up a good practice. The therapist must be able to relate herself to the client sensually and mentally, without either herself or the client

9

becoming involved, and without the client being allowed to become dependent upon her. Therefore the duration of the course of treatment should be quite specific, serving a dual purpose: it also allows the client to feel that her goal is always in sight drawing nearer to being achieved with each successive treatment. This can always be extended and continued.

A high level of intelligence and honesty are necessary so that both the therapist and the client know and understand exactly what the massage or other treatments will accomplish. In this way the therapist protects herself from disillusion and misrepresentation. At the end of the day the therapist can feel satisfied that her work has been honest, worthwhile, and well done. If one form of treatment is found to be unsuitable, it is the therapist who gently guides and suggests another form rather than heavily persuading the client in order to keep a full appointment book. It is then left to the client to make the final decision either to stop, to continue, or to change the course of treatment. In this way she will build up her trust in the therapist and will not feel cheated or let down.

Sensitivity and respect for the body is vital for, although it may represent a mass of fatty tissue, or a connection of bones and muscles from time to time, it does belong to somebody who has a name and a title, so that personal consideration when moving, massaging, and manipulating the client should not be overlooked, especially when the client is dressing and undressing.

Rapport between the therapist and the client should be considered. If for any reason at all the therapist is unable to feel in tune with the client or finds that she has insurmountable personality problems, then she should discuss the situation with her superiors or tactfully transfer treatment to another therapist whose approach to the client may be completely different, so alleviating the source of friction. If she works privately on her own and there is no other solution available then it would be best to discontinue the treatment as soon as possible. One satisfied client's recommendation is worth more than ten dissatisfied customers. Massage is not erotic, although it produces a highly sensual feeling and if a client is suspected of requiring treatment for sexual reasons then it should be stopped immediately and further treatment discontinued. This kind of situation is very rare but requires treatment of the utmost discretion and highest integrity if it ever occurs.

Punctuality whether it is as a student in training or as a qualified practitioner is a habit which should be second nature. Keeping clients waiting and being late for appointments is sheer bad manners, being rarely justifiable. Overbooking of appointments leads to hurried and overlapping treatments, both of which are quite unnecessary. Clients usually prefer to keep the same appointment if possible each day.

Responsibility to colleagues and clients is important and being frequently absent for trivial reasons shows a complete lack of it. Dental appointments should be made out of working hours so that treatments or lectures are not interrupted, continuity is not affected, and the client feels that her beauty therapist is dependable. Personal duties however distasteful should be cheerfully and willingly accepted and carried out without question. In this way the beauty therapist, or potential beauty therapist, builds up her reliability and the reputation of the profession which she represents.

Physical and mental stamina are essential for a job which is absorbing, strenuous, and exacting. As a student she will be required to work physically hard and to apply her mind intelligently to learning the theory. As a qualified therapist she should keep up-to-date with new techniques and modern treatments and should have a sound knowledge of anatomy.

Appearance should be neat and tidy. A uniform should be worn, preferably made out of material which does not attract dirt and can be easily washed. It should give freedom of movement and not be too clinical, although white always looks efficient. Buttons, hooks, and eyes must be replaced immediately when lost and never substituted by safety pins. Dresses and skirts should be well above an even hemline, with nothing showing below, the sleeves should be above the elbow, again with nothing poking below them. Clean teeth, sweet breath, and the regular use of a good deodorant should go without saying. Jewellery should not be worn, though this does not imply removing a wedding ring. A fine ring, such as can be seen in the photographs in this book, has always been permissible; it does not cause pressure or discomfort and cannot be felt during massage. Shoes should be low-heeled for comfort and preferably rubber-soled for quietness and for safety (to prevent slipping on polished floors and when dealing with electricity). Beach sandals and coloured sandals look unprofessional, sloppy, and undignified. Hair if long should be tied well back, otherwise kept neat and tidy if short. Make-up if worn should be natural and well applied. Nails must be short and well manicured, and if nail polish is applied a natural colour should be chosen. Naturally, together with the hands, the nails should be unquestionably scrupulously clean. The beauty therapist should be the ambassador of her profession. Her deportment in her place of work must be calm and quiet. Her own posture should be impeccable, carrying her fresh sparkling uniform proudly. Her attitude should be one of politeness to all those around her including colleagues, superiors, clients, and those who brew the tea and wash the floors. It costs nothing to open a door, or to say 'Good morning' or 'Thank you'.

Etiquette to the doctor if he prescribes treatment or recommends a client to the beauty therapist is shown by carrying out his instructions implicitly. His decision must not be discussed or queried with the client. This applies to treatment prescribed by a superior. If the therapist feels that she cannot comply with the requirements or does not agree about the treatment, then she should have the courtesy to discuss the matter with him and if she still cannot carry out the treatment it would be prudent to give up the case. This applies in the case of a client who knows what treatment she wants. If the therapist feels it is the wrong treatment and cannot conscientiously carry it out she would do best to retract tactfully from the situation. Beauty therapists working in hospitals should always ask the sister-in-charge if it is convenient to visit the wards. She should try to keep the beds tidy and keep out of the way of the hospital routine whilst giving her treatments.

Conversation should be limited to impersonal topics and the therapist should not chatter too much to the client during the course of treatment as it can be tiring. Neither should she inflict her opinions on the client. She should be cheerful but try to dissuade the client from talking too much. However, it is often on the massage couch that the client reveals secrets, personal problems, and worries. These must be kept in strict confidence and whilst listening to the client she should never indulge in gossip with her, or about the client to others. She can be friendly without being familiar but it is generally a mistake to mix personal friendship with professional work. When the client asks for details about the treatment, the therapist must be prepared to explain them in simple terms without long and alarming names. Private medical information should not be disclosed without permission from the source.

Loyalty to colleagues, to superiors, and to the clients is essential to create an atmosphere of warmth, friendliness, and trust. Criticisms of other salons and treatments by the clients is to be discouraged.

Vital Requirements for Massage

The first most important requirement for massage is a pair of well-schooled hands intelligently applied. They should be completely relaxed, warm, and moulded to the part. Some people have a natural ability to relax them more than others but most people are capable of learning good techniques with practice.

Rate of movement should be carried out at a moderately slow speed but this depends upon the effect required.

Rhythm and flow of movement should be even, continuous, and consistent. A good technique depends upon its use throughout all the massage treatments. The rhythm is produced by swaying backwards and forwards from the ankles, knees, and hips.

Stance of the beauty therapist whilst massaging is important to allow her to obtain a good rhythm and freedom of movement. A good stance also helps to avoid back strain and utilizes the body weight correctly. The positions of walk standing when working longitudinally down the length of the muscles, and stride standing when working transversely across the muscles are most frequently used. It is from these positions that the therapist is able to sway rhythmically and fluently whilst massaging, using the body weight effortlessly when required. Stooping not only gives a poor performance, but results in an aching back. The therapist should never lean on the client or on the couch.

Depth of pressure depends upon the area being treated and upon the sensitivity to the tissues of the therapist's hands. She should with experience be able to judge the condition of the tissues, knowing when to decrease or increase the depth accordingly. The back and lower limbs require deeper pressure than that for the neck, chest, and upper limbs. Most clients seem to prefer deep massage but when tissues are delicate, thin, or stretched, and afford little protection to the underlying bones, a light massage is advocated.

Greater depth of pressure is obtained by correct use of body weight transferred through the arms and into the hands. It is not acquired with brute force by pushing harder into the tissues or massaging quickly.

Position of the client should be such that she is well supported, accessible, warm, and comfortable. Clothing should be removed completely if a general body massage is given, and removed from the part locally where required. All the areas of the body which are not being treated should be kept covered with towels and blankets if necessary to ensure warmth. Pillows must support the whole of the limb and not just the area being massaged. This prevents stress and strain on joints and ligaments. For convenience and comfort the client should be either lying or prone lying unless there is some medical reason that necessitates her sitting up. Sometimes the client can be treated sitting at a small table or in a chair but this very much depends upon the area to be massaged. The ability to improvise when a couch is unavailable with the use of pillows and a table is an advantage.

The beauty therapist herself must make the client feel at ease and welcome. Her appearance should be impressive. She should look clean and well groomed, and should accompany the client to the place of treatment and show her out of the salon on completion.

Massage couch or plinth should be the correct working height, sturdy, and with an adjustable back-rest. The therapist should not have to work on one which is either too low causing her to stoop or one which is too high so that she has to stretch, and is unable to use her body weight correctly. It should be wide enough to allow the client to turn over comfortably and yet remain near enough to the therapist without having to be moved closer. The base should be covered with a thin firm mattress and sheet.

Linen should be abundant, always freshly laundered, and scrupulously clean. The client should be covered or wrapped in a sheet and light-weight blanket. Small towels are used for covering locally exposed areas which are not being treated, for covering edges of the sheet and blankets when turned back whilst working on an area, and for placing under parts to afford protection from soiling the bed linen with powders and lubricants. The bed should always be kept as tidy as possible. A plentiful supply of pillows is necessary for the support and comfort of the client.

A trolley on quiet, well-oiled, and smooth-running castors is of great value to be able to wheel equipment easily from one place to another. If there is no table by the couch then the trolley can be laid with the necessary oils, powders, tissues, tape-measure, spare towels, pillows, waste bowl, and everything else that might be required during the course of treatment. It is a good place for a watch which, although necessary, should not be worn on the wrist whilst massaging.

Screens are vital if more than one client is being treated in the same room at once. Again these must be kept in a quiet, smoothly running condition. The curtains on them should be frequently washed and changed as they tend to collect dust.

Electrical machines and all other equipment should be stored neatly out of the way in a corner. Suitable cupboards provided for cosmetics, powders, oils, and suchlike should be kept clean and tidy. Regular stocktaking safeguards shortage of essentials.

Atmosphere and decor of the salon must be relaxing, friendly, and welcoming. It should be tastefully furnished and decorated, making the client feel pleased to be in such surroundings for her treatment. Carpets where possible are warm and deaden sound, but are not always practical round a working space. Here the floors should be kept clean and dry but not highly polished. Although shining floors are preferable because of their look, they can prove to be treacherously dangerous.

Warmth is an important factor and the room must be heated sufficiently, for the body cools quickly when exposed. Good ventilation, however, prevents over-stuffiness and airlessness.

The reception area requires comfortable chairs and up-to-date reading material in case the client has a short wait. Even quiet background music is conducive to a pleasant atmosphere.

Toilets should be within easy reach and as carefully and hygienically maintained as the department, with the usual washing facilities.

A staff room for the therapists is essential. It is in here they can relax, have a coffee, change their clothes, and check their final appearance.

Kitchen facilities that will provide the client with at least coffee or tea are always welcomed.

A wash-basin if possible should be near the couch so that the therapist can wash her hands before and after treatment.

Business Organization

A professional touch does not end with paper qualifications. If rendering a personal service to the public it should be run in a businesslike manner, whether it is a one-man band or not, and many professional people do not know how to run a business. When starting a business it is wise to seek the advice of a solicitor and an accountant on a regular basis so that it is under control at all times.

The receptionist-telephonist should be helpful and courteous with a ready smile to greet the client. She should have the ability to use her initiative in making appointments, taking correct messages, and making decisions without interrupting the beauty therapist at work.

Accounts should be accurately maintained and recorded systematically and daily, so that a complete record of incoming and outgoing moneys can be easily checked.

The tax inspector will require to see books and records of wage deductions, income, and all expenses.

Clients' record cards of treatment must be kept and an efficient filing system maintained. Personal details of the client, such as name, age, marital status, number of children, weight, measurements, are recorded. The name and telephone number of the doctor are taken. Medical history should record major operations, illnesses, or diseases. The date of the client's last visit to the doctor, and the reason, could be quite revealing. Any physical peculiarities must be noted such as birth-marks, scars, bruises, stretch-marks on the skin, or even varicose veins.

If the therapist has any doubt about the health of the client she should ask the client's permission to check with the doctor about the treatment she proposes, which should be recorded. Any untoward effect of the treatment should be noted. The therapist must be on her guard for contra-indications of treatment which might be present or arise, and record anything extraordinary. This not only protects the client from harm but protects the reputation of the beauty therapist. Some establishments prefer their clients to sign a form accepting all responsibility of treatment. However, if no effort has been spared by the beauty therapist in setting a high standard and maintaining it, this should not be necessary.

By thorough and careful examination of the client a general picture of the client's health, fat, muscles, and posture can be built up, and a conclusion can be drawn as to what form the treatment should take. Even if the client only requires half an hour's body massage, she should be given the kind of massage suitable for her type, arrived at by a detailed recorded analysis. Individuality of treatment can be guaranteed by the up-to-date maintenance of efficient record cards. Apart from the benefit to the client in the long run, the standards of the beauty salon will be high and as a business its reputation should grow in esteem.

3. *Manipulations and Massage Technique*

Massage can be defined as a scientific method of manipulating body tissues. It can be performed mechanically by the use of electrical equipment, and manually by hand. The following pages are concerned only with the classification and technique of manual massage. The student must bear in mind that there are different schools of thought on every subject. Massage is no exception but generally speaking classification of manipulations used in massage falls into four main groups. These groups in turn are further sub-divided according to their function and use upon the body tissues. Some French terminology is retained for convenience of description.

Four Groups of Manipulations

1. *Stroking*	Effleurage
	Stroking
2. *Pressure*	Kneading
	Picking up
	Wringing
	Rolling
	Frictions
3. *Percussion*	Hacking
	Clapping
	Beating
	Pounding

19

4. *Shaking*   Vibrations
                                    Shaking

Technique of Manipulations

Part of good technique in massage is to ensure that the client's muscles are completely relaxed. Only if she is relaxed will the massage be truly effective, although, of course, massage itself can be a means to an end by inducing a state of relaxation. However, the client's comfort and support with adequate pillows, blankets, the atmosphere of the salon, and the attitude of the therapist will provide the right medium to work in, and enhance good technique making sure the manipulations are effective.

Stroking Manipulations

EFFLEURAGE

Effleurage is derived from the French word 'effleurer' meaning 'to skim over'. Effleurage can be deep or superficial. The technique for both is identical, except that the pressure varies.

For *deep effleurage* the pressure is finer and deeper. For *light or superficial effleurage* the pressure is superficial and lighter.

TECHNIQUE

It is a stroking movement performed with the whole palmar surface of the hands. It follows the direction of the flow of blood back to the heart, i.e. venous return, and also along the flow of lymphatic vessels ending in a group of lymph glands. On smaller delicate areas such as the toes, fingers, or face the padded palmar surface of the fingertips or thumbs may be used.

The hands may be used alternately, both together, or one may support the area whilst the other is used on its own. Whichever way they are used, the hands must be completely relaxed and moulded to the shape of the limb or part being treated.

The movement must be smooth and rhythmical; pressure is

increased slightly at the end of the stroke, which ends whenever possible in a group of lymph glands, following the course of the veins and lymphatics from the distal end to the proximal end of the limb. The lymph glands for the arm are in the axilla (or armpit); those just above the clavicle are called the supra-clavicular glands. For the face massage, the lymph glands are at the back of the ear; for the leg, they are in the groin, or femoral triangle. (*See* Plates 1 and 2.) Those behind the knee are known as the popliteal lymph glands. At the end of the stroke the hands can glide back with no pressure exerted at all. This maintains continuity and rhythm of movement; contact with the client is unbroken. Some schools of thought prefer to lift the hands off the part at the end of the stroke, and move them back relaxed through the air before commencing again to effleurage. It very often depends on the client's reaction, and if she appears to find the return gliding movement irritating then the latter technique can be employed.

The length of stroke depends upon the part being treated. Effleurage is usually performed slowly, as it is generally a manipulation aimed at the slow circulation.

EFFECTS AND USES OF EFFLEURAGE

1. Promotes the flow of blood in the veins, therefore helping to increase and improve the general circulation.
2. Increases the flow of lymph to the tissues and therefore waste products, amino-acids, fatty acids, and carbon dioxide are more speedily removed into the lymphatic system where they are dealt with and absorbed.
3. Deep effleurage is thought to improve the capillary circulation in the skin, so the nutrition of the skin is aided and the process of healing is assisted, as in a spotty skin or a dry skin. The elasticity of the skin can be improved, as the sebaceous glands secrete more sebum keeping the skin soft and supple.
4. Superficial or light effleurage has a soothing effect on the sensory nerve endings in the skin inducing relaxation in the client.

5. Effleurage helps the client to become accustomed to the therapist's touch. It gives her confidence in the hands of the beauty therapist. It is a manipulation that can provide good continuity in treatment joining up all other manipulations. All massage should begin and end with effleurage. It should be used generously and interspersed frequently throughout all forms of the massage manipulations, helping to emphasize their effects and removing any broken-down tissue products by any of these other manipulations (Plate 3).

Contra-indications

1. Where the limb or area is grossly swollen, as there is a danger of breaking the skin with overstretching.
2. Bad varicose veins where pressure may harm.
3. Hairy areas, as it is uncomfortable.
4. Any area where stretching of the skin could be harmful, such as newly-healed scar tissue, or over-flabby, flaccid muscles.

STROKING

Whilst certain points of technique of stroking are similar to effleurage, it must be entirely distinguished from it as a manipulation.

Stroking can be either: (a) soothing, or (b) stimulating.

TECHNIQUE

It is performed with a relaxed hand which may or may not be moulded to the part. It is entirely independent of the veins and lymphatics, and can be performed in any direction. However, like effleurage, it should be rhythmical. The continuity of the work and the contact should be maintained throughout. Some schools of thought consider it to be effleurage. It can be performed with the whole hand or again with the finger or thumb tips. The dorsum of the hand may be used if desired.

SOOTHING STROKING

It is basically a gentle, slow, and utterly rhythmical manipulation; the touch should be just firm enough for the client to be aware of the stroking, with the whole hand completely relaxed and moulded softly to the part. It is important for the therapist to feel as relaxed and supple as possible to enable this manipulation to be fully effective. The hand is gradually placed on and taken off the client, the return rhythm of the movement in the air being as slow, smooth, and meticulous as the actual stroke, taking the same amount of time to return to the beginning.

Again, like effleurage, one hand may follow the other alternately, both hands may be used together, or the stroking may be done with only one hand whilst the other gently supports the area. The length of the stroke varies according to the area being treated. It can be performed anywhere on the body.

EFFECTS AND USES OF SOOTHING STROKING

1. It soothes the cutaneous nerves and induces relaxation.
2. It can induce sleep and help insomnia.
3. Produces a feeling of restfulness, particularly when performed on the back, from the base of the skull to the bottom of the spine, and is used to relieve tension.
4. The capillaries in the skin contract and swellings can be reduced.
5. Muscle relaxation can be promoted and tension headaches can be relieved by gentle stroking on the brow.
6. Can be used for tense, nervy clients.
7. Stroking can cool down a hot area.

Contra-indications

1. When a client is irritated by stroking.
2. Marked poor circulation such as seen in chilblains and dead white fingers.

STIMULATING STROKING

Performed quickly and vigorously in any direction with the palmar or dorsal aspect of the hand or fingers. Pressure varies according to the treatment as does the length of the stroke.

EFFECTS AND USES OF STIMULATING STROKING

1. The cutaneous nerves are stimulated, therefore a sense of invigoration occurs. Can be used for the treatment of lethargic, obese clients where stimulation of inefficient muscles is required.
2. Involuntary muscle is also stimulated and this manipulation can be used on the abdominal organs to increase their activity if required.
3. Stimulating stroking can stimulate the central nervous system and if used firmly from the base of the head to the bottom of the spine could invigorate and tone up a tired client.
4. Stimulates the glandular activity of the hair follicles, and brisk stroking of the scalp would produce more sebum, so promoting the growth of hair.

Contra-indications

1. Insomnia.
2. Tense, nervous, and excitable clients.
3. Painful areas.
4. Muscle tension.
5. Poor circulation.
6. Clients who dislike stroking.

Pressure Manipulations

The manipulations under this heading are sometimes referred to as petrissage. This word comes from the French 'pétrir' meaning 'to knead'. Kneading incorporates varying manipulations, all of which press the tissues down on to the underlying structures.

Picking up, wringing, and skin rolling incorporate the technique of lifting the tissues away from the underlying structures, namely bone. These three manipulations alone are sometimes referred to as petrissage. They are all essentially pressure manipulations and are used on individual muscles or definite muscle groups, where one end of the muscles to the other is worked upon.

Wringing and skin rolling are manipulations particularly employed for the skin and subcutaneous tissues, such as fat.

Kneading of the abdominal organs has been adapted to suit the area and the function of the organs, so the manipulations simulate the action of peristalsis.

Frictions are stationary pressure manipulations used for localized treatments or small areas where the tissues are pressed down on to the underlying structures.

KNEADING

TECHNIQUE

As with all massage the hands must be supple and relaxed. Kneading has many variations, according to the shape, size, and bulk of the area being treated, so the kneading can be adapted accordingly. But it is *all* kneading. The pressure emphasis is given in the direction of the venous blood return to the heart. The tissues are pressed and relaxed against the underlying bone.

Kneading may, like other manipulations, be performed with one or both hands. It is the whole palmar surface that is used. The muscles are gently squeezed, pressed, and released against the underlying structures. On relaxation of the hands they glide slowly along the muscle or muscle groups being treated. Some authorities consider kneading as a form of petrissage.

Modifications of kneading are considered below. They consist of flat handed, squeezing, circular, and finger kneading as well as ironing (double handed kneading).

FLAT HANDED KNEADING

TECHNIQUE

Sometimes when working on large thin sheets of muscle, such as on the back, squeezing is impossible and the pressure decreases. This is called flat handed kneading.

SQUEEZING KNEADING

In this modification the tissues are squeezed.

EFFECT AND USE

In both squeezing kneading and flat handed kneading there is a slight increase in circulation, used for relaxation, due to its gentle rhythm and superficial effect.

No *contra-indications* are necessary whenever massage is used.

CIRCULAR KNEADING

TECHNIQUE

This manipulation is performed with one or both hands working alternately either side along the length of the limb. The muscles and soft tissues are pressed against the bone in a circular direction. The soft padded surfaces of the palms of the hands and fingers are used, great care being taken that the heel of the hand does not dig into the tissues. Rubbing the skin on bony parts must be avoided by releasing the pressure of the hands when massaging over them. Areas around the shoulder, for example, the coracoid and acromion process of the scapula, the forearm, and the prominent shin bone in the lower leg are particular points to note with this manipulation. However, the pressure should be deep with circular kneading otherwise 'skin rubbing' results if the muscles are not massaged against the bone.

EFFECTS AND USES

1. The main effect is on the muscles. A better blood supply to the muscles is stimulated, therefore they are nourished and fed so helping to maintain elasticity and tone.
2. Improved blood supply will help to carry away fatigue products and carbon dioxide, so refreshing the muscles and helping to alleviate the feeling of stiffness after muscular exertion.
3. When performed rhythmically and slowly down the length of the limb it has a sedative effect and promotes relaxation, also easing away tension and any nervous twitching of muscles.
4. If performed down the length of the spine particularly slowly, a general feeling of restfulness can be obtained and possibly

the client would become so completely relaxed that she would fall asleep.

5. If performed briskly this manipulation can stimulate the muscles and invoke a sense of alertness and well-being on perhaps a rather lethargic client.

6. Because of the pressure of the kneading against the bone, the blood supply to the periosteum is stimulated. Thus, the bone itself is fed and nourished.

7. Kneading is performed on the organs of digestion, which is aided in all its stages by abdominal massage. The end-product of a good digestive system is a glowing healthy skin, always providing that the diet is well balanced in the first place. Kneading on the abdomen can be used to help relieve constipation.

Contra-indications

1. On extremely hairy surfaces.
2. On the abdomen if distended.
3. In cases where massage is completely contra-indicated.
4. Where clients are excessively weak or feeble.

FINGER KNEADING

TECHNIQUE

This is a circular movement performed with the pads of the palmar surfaces of the thumb or first and second fingers localizing the massage (Plate 4). It can be used around the shoulder girdle, down the long back muscles, on small areas such as the face, or soles of the feet or hands. It is similar to frictions but is used mainly for muscles rather than joints. Again the muscle is pressed against the bone and moved in a circular direction.

EFFECTS AND USES

1. Mainly to obtain a localized hyperaemia on small muscles in hands and feet where the larger manipulations would skim over the more intrinsic muscles.
2. Used lightly for more delicate massage as on the face.

3. Used to stimulate the muscles of the arches of the foot and to improve nutrition and tone to these muscles: refreshing and stimulating to someone who has been standing all day long.

IRONING

(Sometimes called reinforced kneading or double handed kneading.)

TECHNIQUE

The technique of ironing is to reinforce one hand on the other so obtaining greater depth, together with body weight (Plate 5). Heavier structures can be moved against the bone, as found in the gluteal region, or on the back.

EFFECTS AND USES

1. Excellent for relieving low back aches where no medical condition exists.
2. Loosens and stretches soft tissues making joints more mobile.
3. If performed slowly and rhythmically can be soothing and relaxing.

PICKING UP

TECHNIQUE

Picking up is quite a stimulating form of petrissage. It can be performed with one or both hands, depending upon the area being treated. The movement should be like all massage, smooth and rhythmic and also continuous from one end of the attachment of the muscle to the other. The technique is to grasp the muscle with the whole hand, making sure that the thumb is completely abducted. The muscle is lifted away from the bone, squeezed, and relaxed again. On relaxation of the part, the other hand, without breaking contact, grasps a fresh area and the movement is repeated in a 'plodding manner' up and down the length of the muscles, or muscle groups. Pinching between the thumb and fingers must be avoided and pressure is given in the upward direction.

If performed with one hand as on the deltoid muscle, then the muscle is grasped either side. Alternatively, one hand can overlap the other with the thumb of one hand overlapping the fingers of the other. The fingers and thumbs of each hand should be straight. This is a lovely manipulation used on the scruff of the neck, an awkward shape and area to manipulate. The muscle group or area to be massaged is treated with the whole hand lifting the tissues at a right angle and away from the underlying bone, is squeezed, and then relaxed again before moving on and a fresh grasp being made.

EFFECTS AND USES

1. Can be used in conjunction with hacking for extremely heavy or fatty areas.
2. Can be used on heavy thick tissues, such as gluteal region or hips where there may not be much mobility of tissues.

WRINGING

TECHNIQUE

The technique of wringing is to lift the structures away from the bone and move them from side to side across the length of the muscle, with the fingers of one hand working with the thumb of the opposite hand (Plate 6). After the tissues have been grasped and stretched, the hands move alternately along the muscles from one end to the other.

EFFECTS AND USES

1. Like all massage it increases the circulation and thus nourishes and feeds the tissues.
2. It is chiefly used on large loose muscle groups so improving tone and elasticity, giving an overall sense of well-being.
3. It is a manipulation which produces heat quickly and absorption is assisted, so that large fatty areas are treated with this manipulation.

SKIN ROLLING

This form of pressure massage (Plate 7) can only be used where there is some underlying hard bone against which the tissues can be pressed and rolled. It affects the skin and subcutaneous tissues.

TECHNIQUE

The technique of skin rolling is to place the hands flat on the area. The skin and soft superficial tissues are grasped firmly between fingers and thumbs and gently rolled backwards and forwards against the thumbs or fingers. It should be performed transversely across the limbs or back, and great care must be taken to ensure comfort of performance.

EFFECTS AND USES

1. Stimulation of blood and skin, increasing nutrition and functions of skin.
2. Used over fatty tissues.
3. This manipulation if performed slowly can be used to induce relaxation. If a brisk rhythm is employed, it can stimulate a client, leaving a sense of invigoration.
4. The skin can be loosened over tight areas making it soft and supple, and also relieving adhesions and releasing tensions. Elasticity of the dermis is improved and maintained.

FRICTIONS

TECHNIQUE

These are small deep movements with much pressure (Plate 8). Before travelling on to a new area, the pressure must be completely released. Frictions are very localized movements performed in a circular or transverse direction with the thumb or fingertips. Circular frictions gradually progress to a maximum depth into the muscle or structures being treated. Transverse frictions maintain a steady and even pressure throughout the movement across the muscle fibres. The fingers must not be hyperextended, especially when working deeply, as this strains the joints of the fingers. It is important to move the skin and superficial structures against the deeper structures with no movement taking place on the surface of the skin. Usually the part needing frictions the most is tender, such as in cases of fibrositis, so care must be taken in application of this manipulation not to cause unnecessary discomfort. Effleurage should be interspersed frequently when frictions are applied.

EFFECTS AND USES

1. Adhesions are broken down, such as stiff joints, or in fibrositic conditions usually found in the back. Localized hyperaemia is produced and this softens the adhesions and helps to bring nourishment to the area.
2. Frictions can loosen and stretch scar tissue.
3. Spinal frictions can produce an invigorating effect through stimulating the spinal nerves leaving the client with a sensation of glowing.
4. Because of the localized hyperaemia, joint structures can be nourished, possible arthritic conditions prevented, and mobility of joints increased and maintained.

Contra-indications

1. All cases of acute inflammation or severe pain.
2. Over joints which are deformed by rheumatoid arthritis.
3. Whenever massage is generally contra-indicated.
4. On bony surfaces.

Percussion Manipulations

These are sometimes referred to as tapotement. They consist of a series of manipulations which strike the body. Both hands are used alternately. The wrists are kept loose and mobile so that the movements produced are light, springy, and stimulating.

HACKING

TECHNIQUE

This is a movement performed with the elbows bent and arms abducted (taken away from the mid-line of the body). The wrists are extended but the fingers should be fairly relaxed (Plate 9). The movement is of pronation and supination of the forearm allowing the ulnar side but dorsal surface of the fifth, fourth, and third fingers to strike the part being treated. The sound should be like falling raindrops and the action should be as sharp and as rapid. If a deeper effect is required, as on the heavy gluteal structures, then the ulnar border only of the hand and fingers can be used. Care must be taken to avoid bony areas and prominences with hacking. Hacking can be performed with the tips of the fingers for more delicate areas such as the face, the movement consisting of flexion and extension of the wrists. This is sometimes known as point hacking, tapping, or digital tapotement.

EFFECTS AND USES

1. If light hacking is performed across the muscle fibres, it can stimulate them to contract without nerve stimulation; therefore hacking can be used to tone up muscles.
2. Its stimulating effect leads to a sensation of invigoration and refreshment to the muscles treated.
3. The client will also experience a glowing sensation due to the increased flow of blood to the muscles, so raising the metabolism due to the increase in temperature.
4. The increased blood supply raises the temperature to the part and hacking can be used for warming up a cold area.
5. A roll of fat can be picked up and hacked with one hand.
6. Hacking tones up the muscular and circulatory systems throughout the body.
7. Hacking down either side of the spine stimulates the spinal nerves and is refreshing.
8. Hacking over the abdominal organs stimulates their actions and aids digestion.

Contra-indications

1. Hacking must never be used over bony areas.
2. On areas which are tending to contract and shorten.

3. On spastic muscles.
4. In cases of excitability or nervousness.
5. In painful conditions.

CLAPPING

TECHNIQUE

This manipulation (Plate 10) is used for the limbs, back, and chest. Again as with all percussion, the wrists must be flexible. Clapping is a movement performed with the palmar surfaces of the hands, which are slightly cupped. The movement of flexion and extension takes place in the wrist. The fingers can either be placed on the part and the heels of the hands are lifted and dropped quickly, or the whole of the cupped hand can be lifted and dropped on to the area being treated. In both instances the hands must spring off the part lightly and quickly, creating a hollow, cupping sound.

EFFECTS AND USES

1. Increases blood flow to the skin and so improves condition of skin.
2. Increases blood flow to the lungs in the thorax, therefore there is a better interchange of gases in the lung capillaries. In turn, more oxygen will be carried to the tissues of the body and the gaseous waste products exhaled.
3. Loosens mucus to hollow organs, such as the lungs.
4. Because of the increase of activity of the lung tissue their resistive powers to infection can be said to be increased.
5. Increases the circulation of the area treated and causes increased nutrition and a sensation of warmth.
6. This manipulation can be used again over fatty tissue.

Contra-indications

1. The same as for hacking.
2. Where the client has had tuberculosis of the lungs, to the chest only.
3. Never applied over abnormally contracted muscles.

BEATING

TECHNIQUE

Beating is a heavier manipulation similar to clapping, but it is performed with a loosely clenched fist, so that the dorsal part of the fingers strike the client and the heel of the hand comes into contact with the part to be treated. The hands again work alternately, but one only can be used, e.g. over the sacrum or liver.

POUNDING

TECHNIQUE

This is another form of heavy percussion. It is a movement similar to hacking, the loosely clenched fist striking the part to be treated with the ulnar border of the hand.

EFFECTS AND USES OF BEATING AND POUNDING

1. Used over the liver they will stimulate cell activity. More bile will be produced and therefore sluggish digestion aided. This in turn shows its improved effects in the tissues of the body.
2. Can be used to stimulate the nerves in the sacral area. This in turn helps to quicken peristalsis, improve digestion, and relieve constipation.
3. Can be used on areas where the subcutaneous fat is dense and heavy, so helping to soften the adipose tissue.
4. Imparts a healthy glow to the part being massaged and tones up the muscles.
5. With each striking movement the muscles first contract and then relax as the fingers are removed from the body. Muscle activity is increased with this manipulation.
6. All other effects as for hacking and clapping.

Contra-indications

1. Where tissues are thin and delicate.
2. Over bony areas to prevent bruising.

3. In cases of general weakness and where the client is excessively thin, as these manipulations are far too heavy.
4. All other contra-indications as for hacking and clapping.

Shaking Manipulations

VIBRATIONS

TECHNIQUE

Vibrations are a fine trembling-like movement performed with one or both hands, using either the whole palmar surface or the fingertips. The movement consists of small quick flexions and extensions at the fingers and wrist joints. The therapist's arm and hands must be completely relaxed as it is a tiring manipulation, and will not be effective if tension in the operator's muscles is produced. The vibrations can be *static*, i.e. performed in one place, or they can be *running* where the hand or fingertips travel over the part whilst still vibrating. They can be fine, or coarse and more vigorous.

EFFECTS AND USES

1. Scar tissue can be loosened.
2. Fine vibrations have a sedative effect and can be used over nerves and nerve centres to relax a client.
3. Relieves flatulence in the abdominal organs.
4. Coarse vibrations are stimulating.
5. Vibrations performed down the spinal column with the fingertips will stimulate a lethargic client and produce a sensation of alertness and refreshment.

Contra-indications

1. Coarse vibrations as for tapotement where all cases for stimulation are undesirable.
2. Fine vibrations are contra-indicated where massage in all forms is contra-indicated.

SHAKING
TECHNIQUE

Shaking is similar to vibrations, being performed with relaxed hands. It is a shaking movement of the hands moving the part up and down, or from side to side, or in and out.

EFFECTS AND USES

1. The same effects as for percussion.
2. Loosens mucus in lungs.
3. Stimulates liver cells.
4. If used to shake the limbs, the bone marrow is said to be stimulated thus increasing output of red blood corpuscles and therefore enriching the blood stream.
5. Can increase the vitality and functional activity of the abdominal and thoracic organs; therefore it is of great value to the body generally.

Contra-indications

As for percussion.

Summary of Effects of Massage

All the various manipulations of massage have to some extent the same effect. The chief effect of massage is definitely on the circulation and, in turn, by this manner can influence the various tissues and organs of the body. There is little effect on the activity of the muscles and therefore the tone, which can only be improved effectively by active exercise. Correcting faulty eating habits by well-balanced diets is the best means for reducing fatty tissue. However, each manipulation has its own special effect on some particular tissue, and the student should learn which manipulation to apply for the kind of effect she is hoping to bring about.

Effleurage chiefly affects the flow of lymph, the blood back to the heart and the circulation. It is useful in cases of fatigue, aids absorption of waste and broken-down products, helps healing processes, and increases the nutrition of the tissues. It is used for nourishing the skin, so improving its functions.

Stroking affects mainly the nerve endings in the skin. It is useful in relaxing or stimulating a client according to whether soothing or stimulating stroking is used.

Pressure manipulations stimulate muscle or muscle groups, increasing their circulation and so improving nutrition, helping to restore tired function and improve tone, especially after exercise when stiffness can be alleviated. Used most frequently in an abdominal massage, improving the functioning of the abdominal organs.

Wringing and skin rolling is used especially on adipose tissue to soften and break down fatty masses. Good for loosening muscles and adherent skin, maintaining elasticity.

Picking up is often applied to muscle bellies and to a lesser degree to the tendons.

Frictions bring about a local hyperaemia and quite definitely aid absorption of inflammatory products. Mostly used around joints, so increasing mobility, also in the long muscles of the back and around all tender spots on the back, breaking down tension areas causing pain. Can be used to loosen scar tissue and stimulate the the spinal nerves. Care must be taken not to cause a deadening sensation with too much pressure, unless specifically required.

Percussion is used to stimulate nerves and muscles and give a feeling of increased tone. It also stimulates nerves, leaving a general exhilarating and glowing sensation. Again, too much percussion on one spot can deaden the area. It can be used to soften fatty tissue for weight reduction. Combined with picking up, hacking can help to break down subcutaneous fat. Also used in loosening mucus in the lungs, therefore promoting a better gaseous interchange and allowing more oxygen to be taken to the muscles. It also stimulates deep organs in the abdomen to better functioning.

Vibrations and shakings especially affect nerves and organs. According to the effect required and manipulation used, they can soothe or stimulate nerves, thus producing a relaxation of the client, or invigoration. They also loosen mucus in the lungs and stimulate the cells of the abdominal organs. Useful for constipation, sluggish liver, and poor digestion.

Psychological Effects of Massage

Massage has been endowed with powers of magic beyond all imagination, and it is as well to bear in mind its limitations. However, the psychological effects produced are unlimited and cannot be underestimated by any manner of means. The marvellous tonic effect of massage is not only confined to the healthiest and most normal person, but its value has been recognized by psychiatrists and doctors. A beauty care service organized by the Red Cross has spread up and down the country, to help people in psychiatric wards, and long-term patients in other hospitals throughout the country.

It is necessary for the therapist to understand that many benefits received from massage are physiologically impossible without long-term and regular treatment. This, on no account, means that its value is less. Health, both physical and mental, is the basis of beauty and in the busy average day when all systems are go, tensions mount and relaxation is impossible. These tensions of the mind and body begin to show on the face and in the body, which ages and deteriorates. Men and women alike have little time to spare for relaxation at home, and very often there is nowhere to go where their peace remains undisturbed, even if they have time.

So they visit the beauty salons to escape the hectic city life and enter the serene and pleasant atmosphere that should welcome them. Minor aches and pains caused by nervous tensions can be soothed and massaged away as the sense of relaxation seeps over the body. A glowing sensation of well-being is promoted after a well-executed massage.

Some clients who feel they are aging fast may not look younger after treatment but feel completely rejuvenated. Some clients, young or old, need the help of massage to encourage them to stick to rigid diets, especially if they feel that the fatty tissues are being softened and broken down more quickly. Other clients merely want to avail themselves of the luxury of being pampered, soothed, and being made to feel beautiful by massage; they enjoy spending time in having their bodies looked after and enhanced. Others like the pleasant sensory effect that massage can give.

Perhaps, during the course of treatment, a client needs the comfort of a sympathetic and willing ear to listen to her troubles. A client may need reassurance about her figure, face, or age and may feel that massage does much to benefit her in this way.

Many clients really feel that aches and pains are cured with massage; perhaps it is because the tensions causing the aches and pains have been reduced by a relaxing massage and very often disappear. The increased circulation does help to relieve pain also. Some clients need to feel stimulated and alert and a brisk massage will invoke a sensation of invigoration.

Feeling refreshed, invigorated, glowing, and marvellous for whatever reason at the end of a treatment of massage is the keynote that it has been successful. An experienced masseuse will recognize immediately what it is that a client requires, and she will endeavour to provide the conditions and massage necessary for such a treatment. Remember that beauty radiates outwards from within. Psychologically the client benefits by massage because she simply feels it is doing her good. She feels healthier and in turn looks healthier.

Even if massage had no physical benefits whatsoever, the beauty salons would still be full of people requiring massage for the wonderful sensation that it produces.

General Contra-indications of Massage

1. In recent injuries and any condition that requires medical supervision.
2. Tumours or unrecognizable lumps.
3. Over varicose veins or phlebitis or thrombosis.

4. In acute inflammatory conditions.
5. Rheumatoid arthritic joints.
6. Swollen ankles due to other causes than long periods of standing.
7. Grossly swollen limbs.
8. In pregnancy.
9. Immediately prior to and during a period to the abdomen or sacral areas.
10. Neuritis and neuralgia.
11. Acutely painful areas.
12. When the temperature is raised.
13. Skin diseases.
14. Over especially hairy area due to discomfort.
15. Abdominal massage in cases of diarrhoea, high blood pressure, and hernia.
16. In cases of lung disease.
17. Over unhealed and recently healed wounds and scars.
18. In the area of boils or carbuncles or round septic conditions.
19. Haemophilia where a client might bleed easily if accidentally bruised.
20. In older clients with a tendency to arterio-sclerosis (hardening of the arteries) a vigorous massage would be contra-indicated.
21. Loss of skin sensation.
22. Low blood pressure.
23. Glandular obesity.

Lubricants, Oils, Powder, and Massage Creams

As far as the therapist is concerned, if she is skilled enough and her technique of massage perfected to a fine art, she should not need to use any form of lubricant or powder. However, if it should be necessary from her point of view to use an aid of this kind, it should be used as sparingly as possible.

Sometimes the client requests that certain oils or creams are used, according to the claims of the beauty preparations, and she will feel that her massage has added value if the benefits are massaged into the skin and body. Whatever emollient is used it should always be applied to the hands of the therapist first and not directly on to the client.

Oil—olive oil softens and nourishes the skin and subcutaneous tissues. It will lubricate a dry skin and enable the masseuse to stretch the skin without tearing or skin rubbing so that she can massage deeper into the tissues. This in turn makes the skin more supple. If deep frictions are given it is advisable to use oil in order to obtain maximum penetration. It is no use trying to disguise wet, sticky hands by using oil, for they will merely slide off the client, producing an irritating and unsatisfactory massage. Essential oils are becoming widely used in beauty therapy.

Powder—the finest of powders should be used and preferably one with the most innocuous smell. Fine French chalk or even a brand-named baby powder is suitable. The therapist's hands should be powdered: never under any circumstance should the therapist powder the client as though using salt and pepper on a bag of chips. The powder is of no benefit to the client, but purely to the hands of the operator, who may be a bit sticky. If the skin is dry, powder will only irritate the condition. Keep the use of powder down to a minimum. Flapping it around in the air creates a dusty atmosphere and gets in the eyes and nose of the client.

Soap, oil, and hot water can be discreetly used in cases where the client has dirty or scaly patches of skin, until the condition is alleviated. Sometimes the soles of the feet are neglected, or on a wet rainy day the shoe dyes soak through to the skin.

Cold massage cream can be used over hairy surfaces which can then be massaged satisfactorily. Cream can be used in the same manner and for the same reason as powder. Creams are usually more readily absorbed into the skin than oil. Again, the importance of applying it first to the hands of the masseuse cannot be stressed too strongly. Always use extra towels when applying particularly greasy lubricants. Excessive lubricants at the end of the massage can be wiped off with eau-de-cologne or surgical spirit, according to the preference of the client.

Hand Exercises

Relaxation and suppleness of the hands and joints of the hands is most important. Exercises should be practised daily until all the joints are free and mobile. Both hands should be able to work equally well. They should be well manicured, smooth, and warm.

Practise the following exercises before attempting to massage:

1. Quickly make a fist clenching and stretching out the fingers.
2. Roll the thumbs round and round, first one way, then the other.
3. Roll each finger round.
4. Stretch each finger separately and then together.
5. Place index fingers and thumbs together and try to stretch them in a straight line.
6. Separate the fingers slowly and quickly.
7. Bend the fingers straight over from the metacarpo-phalangeal joint (knuckle) and back as far as they will go.
8. Flap the wrists up and down, from side to side, and in a circle until they feel completely loose, relaxed, and both moving equally.
9. Bend the elbows and turn the palms first to the floor and then to the ceiling quickly in pronation and supination.
10. Shake wrists again together and then alternately.
11. Palms together, elbows out at the sides, stretch back the wrists in a prayer position.
12. Kneading a soft ball.
13. Whole arm and shoulder shaking.
14. Circling wrists round and round.

Hints for Practising Technique

1. *Develop* sensitivity by practising feeling the shapes of different objects with the eyes closed. Anything will do at any time and any place. Then practise feeling the shape and size of the tissues to be massaged by relaxing the hands completely and drawing them gently over the areas and contours of the body.

2. *Use spirit* and cologne on moist, sticky hands. Damp hands are a disadvantage in massage but, as confidence grows, tenseness resulting in perspiring hands disappears.

3. *Practise* hacking, clapping, beating, and pounding on a hard wooden surface until it can be performed with ease for ten minutes at a time painlessly.

4. *Use hand cream* to keep the hands smooth and soft.

5. *Wash hands* frequently and always before and after a massage.

6. *Soak cold hands* under hot tap prior to massaging, although they do soon warm up and cold hands are often an advantage in massage as they rarely become sticky during treatment.

7. *Depth and strength* of manipulation is varied by the correct use of body weight. Practise the changing of the two most important positions of the feet until it becomes second nature to swivel from one into the other.

8. *Practise* the smooth change from one manipulation to another for good continuity.

9. *Use music* to practise rhythm and speed of manipulations.

10. *Try to massage* a client on a plinth or massage couch suitable to the therapist's own requirements. If the couch is too low, stand further away and bend from the hips keeping the back straight. If the masseuse works with a bent back she will get backache and the treatment will be poor.

4. *The Physiological Effects of Massage*

Effects on the Muscles

When muscles work, they need a greater supply of oxygen, and more waste products are produced. The waste products can accumulate when the muscles are resting, and stiffness results. If muscles are massaged the blood supply is increased. This increased circulation not only feeds the muscle tissue, but brings with it oxygen and absorbs the waste products. Muscles are kept in tone and functional power with massage. However it is important to realize the limitations of massage, and to understand that nothing can have the same value as active exercise. An athlete will always feel refreshed after great muscular exertion when massaged, as the acceleration of the blood will help to carry away the toxic products formed in the muscles during strenuous exercise.

Due to an increased production of heat because of the improved blood supply to the muscles, the whole body will feel warmer and the temperature can be raised. So it can be seen that a vigorous massage of the muscles will produce in them a warm glow throughout the body.

Increase and improvement in tone causes an increase in elasticity and extensibility. Tense and short muscles can be relaxed and stretched with massage. This factor can be made use of when correcting postural faults. Very often with bad posture the flexor groups of muscles tend to shorten and contract gaining tone. The extensor muscles become over-stretched and lose tone. For instance, tight pectoral muscles across the chest could be greatly massaged, bearing relaxation in mind, whilst the back extensor muscles are given a vigorous and stimulating treatment. This would help to stretch and relax the hollow tight chest, and strengthen up the rounded back.

Again, bearing in mind that the muscular system is really dependent upon active exercise for its greatest increase in tone and size, massage can be a valuable accessory to their normal functioning. Muscles work over joints and, if the mobility of the joints is impaired by any kind of adhesions, then the function of the muscles will in turn suffer, as full-range movement will be prevented. Therefore massage, such as frictions, around and into joints will help to prevent adhesions, or loosen and stretch them. Mobilizing the joints in this way will indirectly help the movement of the muscles, enabling weak muscles to move more easily and increase their range. Weakened muscles, due to long periods of disuse, can be benefited by massage and more readily returned to normal, than if left unused and unaided.

The alternate pressure and relaxation on each muscle fibre causes an increased circulation to it. Blood is said to flow three times more quickly through a muscle which has been massaged. This improved blood supply increases nutrition to the muscle fibre, and in turn of the whole muscle and muscle groups.

Kneading and all other forms of pressure manipulations, including effleurage, can improve muscle tone and delay wasting away of muscles through disuse. Although beauty therapists do not practise heart massage, it should be remembered that the heart is a muscle too, and many lives have been saved by massage to this special muscle.

Effects on the Bones and Joints

Pressure against the periosteum stimulates the blood circulation to the bones. This feeds and nourishes the bone itself and also the joints in the neighbouring area. Indirectly, massage to the muscles of the body can affect the direction of bone growth. Bone tends to grow in the direction of the least pressure. The flexed group of muscles exert the strongest pressure and force on the bones. If the flexors are massaged to help them relax in cases of tension and the extensor group of muscles stimulated by massage then the direction of the growth of bone could be influenced in this manner by massage with regular treatment. Mild postural deformities can be helped and possibly prevented, especially in young people.

Maintaining and increasing the mobility of joints is another effect of massage when regularly applied. Certain manipulations can help to prevent adhesions and stiffness in joints improving and maintaining their full range of movement.

Effects on the Circulatory and Lymphatic System

Because the veins contain so many valves, regurgitation or back flow is impossible and the flow of venous blood always moves towards the heart. The smaller veins on the surface of the skin link up to the larger ones and eventually to the two large venous trunks which return the blood to the right side of the heart. This direction of flow is called 'centripetal'. The superficial veins are very easily palpated and it takes only slight pressure to empty them. So it can be seen that light superficial effleurage can affect the flow of blood very easily and possibly help the work of the heart, although it is doubtful that massage can directly affect the circulation in the arteries or the heart itself. The improvement of the blood flow in the veins is made use of in massage by interspersing effleurage freely, throughout all forms of massage, in order to carry away waste products, toxins, and carbon dioxide efficiently and quickly into the blood stream. In return for the quickened venous circulation, oxygen and all nutriments are brought back by way of the arteries. Gentle stroking produces a contraction of the walls of the capillaries in the skin which has a cooling effect on the body.

Effleurage and kneading accelerates also the lymphatic circulation. Kneading squeezes the lymph from the lymph spaces, and the effleurage moves it on to the nearest lymph glands. Fresh lymph seeps through the walls of the capillary blood vessels to feed the tissues, absorbing products of fatigue and wear and tear of the areas. If there is a local infection then the lymph fluid will help to pass it on to the lymph glands which will become swollen and sore in an effort to fight the germs, although massage is contra-indicated for local infections. When the lymphatic circulation becomes stagnant then the area becomes grossly swollen. This swelling can be considerably relieved by massage, providing there is no condition present which requires medical supervision.

Effects on the Lungs

The condition of the lungs can be improved by massage. Mobilizing the joints of the thorax, strengthening and improving the tone of the respiratory muscles by massage indirectly will help with airing the lungs. Such manipulations as percussion will have a direct effect on the lung tissue. Not only will the circulation to the bronchioles be improved, thus feeding the tissues and helping to maintain elasticity, but any mucus or foreign particles, if present, can be dislodged with such manipulations. With the increased nutrition to the lung tissue, gaseous interchange is also increased, ridding the body of carbon dioxide and replenishing it with oxygen. There is a possibility that massage to large muscle groups producing an increased circulation and combustion in the tissues will increase the amount of carbon dioxide in them. This in turn could cause a need for a deeper and more thorough inspiration and expiration so effecting movement of the lungs.

Effects on the Skin

Any massage manipulation affects the skin which has many functions. To a certain extent, like all the other systems, these functions are made more active by massage. Circulation to the skin is improved and the secretory glands, so nourished by fresh blood, produce more sebum. This in turn makes the skin soft and supple and increases its resistance to infection. More sweat is produced by the activated sudiferous (sweat) glands which excrete urea and other waste products. By massage, the top dead layer of skin cells can be rubbed off. This enables the skin to breathe more easily, again improving the condition of the skin, and allowing tissue respiration to be assisted, imparting an overall healthy glow. If the top horny layer of skin is massaged away, its functions of absorption and protection will be performed much more efficiently. In the skin too lie the peripheral nerve endings. With massage the sensory nerve endings can either be soothed, or stimulated, according to the type of massage manipulations employed and required for treatment.

Effects on Adipose Tissue

There is little, if any, effect that occurs when massaging the fatty tissues of the body. Fat requires a chemical reaction to take place and necessitates the presence of certain enzymes before it can be broken down or metabolized. However, the following theories have all been propounded and it is still widely believed that fat can be broken down with massage despite the scientific facts which appear to prove otherwise.

When fatty masses are treated by massage, the heat in the fatty tissue is produced more quickly by the increased circulation. This latter aids absorption of the fat, and the increased metabolism of the tissues helps to burn it up. Also it is believed that the fatty globules may be released by massage and spread over a larger area for absorption into the lymphatic system.

Therefore dense areas of firm solid fat can be softened and, when massage is combined with a scheme of weight-reducing exercises plus a slimming diet, its effect will be greatly increased. If massage breaks down fatty tissue in local areas without diet and exercises it will be merely displaced and deposited elsewhere in the body. Sometimes tissue fluids are trapped around the fat globules, making fat reduction by dieting alone, a hard task. Massage with its effect of pushing the tissue fluids along and speeding up the flow of circulation can help in reducing oedema caused by fat globules retaining the fluid. Again reduction of tissue fluids makes for easier absorption of adipose tissue as it becomes more available for combustion in the body metabolism.

There are many sceptical schools of thought about the effect of breaking down fatty tissue by massage. The student and therapist should bear in mind that to be most effective the massage must be performed regularly and vigorously. For weight reduction, massage combined with diet and exercise is the ideal combination.

Effects on the Nerves

The vigorous manipulations of massage, namely vibrations, frictions, and percussion, generally have a stimulating and invigorating effect on the nerves of the body. Pressure on nerves sufficient to block out impulses can have a deadening effect, and will temporarily relieve pain. It is a natural instinct to press a painful spot, so relieving pain. Percussion such as hacking may have a reflex effect on them, and in turn, because they are mechanically stimulated in this way, many tissues and organs in the body can be influenced to function more efficiently. For example, if the secretory nerves of the stomach are stimulated, the stomach will produce more digestive juices to aid digestion. Another effect of massage is the soothing one which it has upon the nervous system gaining relaxation either locally or for the whole body. Slow rhythmic manipulations can produce sleep by causing the nerves to respond reflexly to this gentle stimulation. Massage of the head, neck, shoulders, and back can be hypno-tically relaxing. This can revive tired nerves suffering from exhaustion and revitalize them. In the same way as has already been mentioned brisk vigorous massage on the head and back will stimulate the central nervous system.

Effects on the Abdominal Organs

Kneading of the alimentary tract affects the involuntary muscle wall and simulates its action, namely that of peristalsis. Peristaltic movement is increased by the pressure exerted on the stomach wall, small intestine, and colon. If the manipulations are per-formed quickly, then stimulation of the muscular abdominal wall results. The circulation to this area is also increased.

Shaking and hacking are used over these organs to increase their vitality and function. By stimulating them with this form of percussion, more secretions are produced and digestion will be aided. Vibrations can soothe the nerves of the alimentary tract relieving flatulence and intestinal spasm (felt sometimes as 'butterflies').

Gentle stroking and kneading of the colon is said to help mechanically the flow of its contents.

Stimulating stroking over the organs of digestion has an effect reflexly on the involuntary muscle, and is used when an invigorating effect is required. Massage of the liver increases and stimulates cell activity. By slow deep manipulations the liver cells produce more bile which is stored in the gall bladder until required.

Metabolism and Beauty

The ability by which the body is able to convert food and other substances into suitable energy to its own use is called metabolism. It includes the taking in of food and oxygen which repairs broken-down and used tissues. The foodstuffs are worked upon by the different juices of the digestive system, broken down, and then, when digested, are absorbed and rebuilt in the body's metabolic processs. Chemical reactions taking place in the tissues, to produce the necessary energy for muscle actions, generation of nerve centres, and for all the other functioning of the different systems of the body, are included as part of metabolism. If food substances are not correctly metabolized then certain diseases can occur when chemical reactions are affected. Obesity, gout, and diabetes are some examples of metabolic diseases. Minor health ailments caused through incorrect metabolism for whatever reason can have a marked effect on inward and outward beauty. Take someone who is overweight but not suffering from a severe case of obesity that needs medical attention. Not only does she (or he) feel miserable if she looks unsightly but her eating of the wrong kind of foodstuffs may well cause the digestive organs to rebel and produce indigestion. This in turn, apart from the aesthetic point of view, could register as pain on the face, possibly causing poor posture and lethargy: an ideal case for beauty treatment.

There are many people with such beauty problems, not requiring medical attention, who find their way into the beauty salons. Those who are lucky enough not to require anything more than the pure luxury that the beauty salons can give are few and far between. Spots, overweight, greasy skins, dry skins, flatulence, poor posture, and cramp are but a few of the conditions discussed with the beauty therapist. Many such problems arise from faulty metabolism for one reason or another.

One of the paths to beauty is through the stomach, and the digestive system can be considered as its heart. It is from here that the metabolism of the foodstuffs begins, as already been stated, and poor metabolism can affect the inward and outward vitality of the body health.

All the finest clothes and purest cosmetics, however skilfully applied, cannot disguise for long the malfunctioning of any of the systems of the body, particularly the digestive system.

Massage where it is not contra-indicated is one of the vital tools in helping to correct the symptoms of a faulty metabolism, promoting health and beauty throughout all the systems of the body.

5. *Order and Method of Work*

Preparation and Procedure

SALON

Before the client arrives for her massage treatment the therapist should check the client's name, record card, and time of appointment so that she can be absolutely ready on her arrival. All necessary equipment required to be used during the massage should be prepared beforehand. This includes not only the layout of the trolley with its talcum powder, oil, massage cream, tissues, and all materials which may be used during the treatment, but also spare towels, and pillows to prevent the therapist from unnecessary breaks in the massage itself because she has forgotten something. The continuity and flow of the treatment cannot be over-emphasized. If the therapist must turn to reach for something from the trolley, one hand if possible should remain in gentle contact with the client to maintain continuity. If the masseuse is required to leave the client and break off the treatment completely then the client should be covered with a towel and a courteous apology made. Scrupulously clean linen and blankets should greet the eye of the client. No one likes to feel that she is lying between second-hand sheets or that the gowns and towels are not freshly laundered. A gown into which the client can change should be ready. If screens are necessary to ensure privacy they should be arranged in readiness around the couch. The room must be warm and an adequate supply of blankets provided, as muscles which are cold cannot be relaxed.

Lighting should be checked to see that it is not too glaring, and noise must be kept to a minimum.

THERAPIST

The beauty therapist must wear a clean fresh overall and check that her hair is tidy, make-up not too striking, and that her personal freshness is ensured by the liberal use of good deodorants. She should remove any rings, bracelets, or necklaces. Before the massage begins she should wash and dry her hands.

CLIENT

The client must be greeted warmly and directed personally to the couch or cubicle to be used. If it is her first visit to the salon a friendly chat with the client will put her at her ease. During this time the record card can be filled in with all relevant information about the client, including the name, address, and telephone number of her doctor. The treatment can be discussed and the therapist can also ascertain that she has no medical conditions present which would contra-indicate body massage or any other form of treatment. When the client is relaxed she can be asked to change into the gown and lie on the couch. The therapist should then examine the client for scars, varicose veins, and visible contra-indications which would modify the massage. If required the client should be weighed and measured.

POSITION OF CLIENT AND BEAUTY THERAPIST

When settling the client comfortably, make sure that she is in such a position as to require the minimum amount of disturbance for the whole treatment. Depending upon which part of the body is to be massaged and whether the treatment is localized or generalized, so her position will vary. If only the arms are to be massaged then she could quite easily be treated comfortably sitting up. If the whole body is to be massaged it is a good idea to position her in lying either prone or supine according to requirements. Ample support from pillows is essential however the client is placed, for her maximum support and comfort. As the body soon cools down when exposed, plenty of blankets will ensure warmth. It is important to take into consideration before asking the client to relax completely, that she is not settled too far away from the operator on the couch. This would result in ineffective massage, apart from strain on the beauty therapist's arms and back. Incorrect positioning of the therapist or client can only result in poor technique. The therapist must place her feet in such a position as to be able to pivot freely from walk standing, which is with one foot in front of the other, into stride standing, which is with both feet a few inches apart and parallel during the massage (*see* Chapter 10 for positions). When working longitudinally down the length of the muscle fibres the therapist generally stands in walk standing position, but when massaging transversely across the the muscle fibres she swivels into stride standing. If her foot positions are incorrect, then body weight in the massage is thrown out of balance and once again, because the rhythm, depth, and smoothness are affected, technique is poor and the massage can only be bad. Apart from the client suffering and losing out, the therapist will no doubt begin to develop a chronic backache as well as a diminishing clientèle if, throughout a hard day's work, her positioning has been wrong.

TENSION

It is because so many people are tense and unrelaxed that they have found their way onto the couch of the masseuse, for massage is a good relaxer. But total relaxation of the client does not only depend upon the benefits derived from the massage itself. To be truly effective on the muscles and tissues of the body, the mind should be completely relaxed. Therefore, from the first moment of contact with the client, the therapist must create a peaceful, calm, unhurried, and reassuring atmosphere. Even if she is only making the appointment, her attitude and tone of voice can do much to make the client feel welcome and wanted. Most clients feel a little nervous, apprehensive, and shy on their first visit to the salon. Massaging taut muscles is a difficult and tiring job, even for the most experienced masseuse. Much can be achieved to aid relaxation of the client if the therapist herself has learnt the art of relaxation.

Naturally the massage itself cannot be good if the therapist's hands are stiff and unrelaxed because of her own personal irritations and tensions. A musician, too, gives a poor performance if he is unrelaxed and his fingers are wooden. There are opera singers who are so afraid of being emotionally upset before an engagement that they will not talk to anyone for forty-eight hours before a performance in case their voice is affected. One can hardly consider a massage in quite the same light but relaxation of the therapist plays a dramatic role in performance and effect. When the therapist puts on her overall she must leave behind her own problems. This applies when she takes it off again at the end of the day. Work finished, hands washed for the last time, and overall discarded, the client's personal problems must be left behind. This is essential for the mental hygiene of the beauty therapist and ultimately ensures that she starts each day vitally refreshed. Chapter 11 describes some general relaxation methods which the beauty therapist can practise and teach.

The first steps towards a successful treatment will have begun when the beauty therapist appears, relaxed and unhurried, paying particular attention to the sounds around and ensuring that equipment is not clattered about. Use of the client's name and a pleasant smile ushering her gently to her cubicle will also invoke a further sense of confidence in the client, which encourages a totally relaxed state of mind and body, ready for the treatment to begin.

Order and Method of General Massage

Massage like baking a cake has certain basic ingredients and simple rules to follow. Once these are grasped, they can be adapted to suit any type of person on any part of the body, for whatever treatment is required. General massage is a complete massage of all parts of the body, except the face and head. A general massage lasts for about sixty minutes. The work throughout should be smooth and very rhythmic; the hands must follow and mould to the contours of the parts at all times. Break in continuity should be avoided, and contact maintained always. Where it is necessary to work with one hand, the other should be used to support the part of limb worked upon and not left to dangle idly around, or used as a leaning prop on the client. When the client needs to be moved, it should be simply and quickly done without fuss or flapping of blankets, towels, or sheets.

The rate of massage depends upon the kind of treatment given. In practising technique a moderate rate should be adopted. This can be speeded up or slowed down as required, bearing in mind that a total of sixty minutes only gives a minimum amount of massage to any one area in a general body massage.

The work throughout should be deep, unless contra-indicated; body weight for the back and lower limbs is essential. Walk and stride standing are the positions most frequently used by the beauty therapist.

Programme for full General Body Massaage lasting 60 minutes

FIRST POSITION

The client lies supine (face upwards), pillows supporting head, back of neck, and under knees.

ORDER OF MASSAGE

1. Right arm.
2. Left arm.
3. Neck and chest.
4. Right leg.
5. Left leg.
6. Abdomen.

SECOND POSITION

The client lies prone (face downwards), pillows supporting face and neck and shoulders, under front of abdomen and hips, under front of ankles.

ORDER OF MASSAGE

1. Back, neck, and shoulders.
2. Buttocks.

N.B. All areas not being massaged should be covered up, and the client should not be required to move more than is necessary.

PROGRAMME FOR ARMS (UPPER EXTREMITY OR LIMB)

1. Effleurage of whole arm, covering whole arm three times.
2. Kneading upper arm three times.
3. Wringing and picking up of upper arm three times.
4. Finger kneading round elbow joint twice.
5. Kneading of forearm and hand twice.
6. Petrissage to forearm twice.
7. Finger and thumb kneading to forearm twice.
8. Finger kneading to wrist and tendons of hand joints, fingers, and palms twice.
9. Percussion to whole arm twice.
10. Effleurage three times.

Time for each arm about five minutes.

PROGRAMME FOR CHEST AND NECK

1. Effleurage down sides of neck and across chest to cover three times.
2. Flat handed kneading twice.
3. Finger kneading twice.
4. Light hacking twice.
5. Effleurage three times.

Time for chest about five minutes.

PROGRAMME FOR LEGS (LOWER EXTREMITY OR LIMB)

1. Effleurage of whole leg covering four times.
2. Kneading to thigh four times.

3. Wringing and picking up to thigh four times.
4. Effleurage round knee twice.
5. Finger and thumb kneading round knee twice.
6. Kneading to lower leg twice.
7. Wringing and picking up to calf twice.
8. Finger kneading to anterior tibial muscles twice.
9. Finger and thumb kneading all round ankle and Achilles tendon twice.
10. Stroking round ankle and foot twice.
11. Deep kneading to foot four times.
12. Finger and thumb kneading to foot and toes twice.
13. Percussion to whole leg once.
14. Effleurage four times.

Time taken for each leg about seven minutes.

PROGRAMME FOR ABDOMEN (ABDOMINAL WALL)

1. Effleurage or stroking three times.
2. Kneading three times.
3. Wringing and picking up twice.
4. Hacking three times.
5. Vibrations once.
6. Stroking three times.

Time taken for abdomen about seven minutes.

PROGRAMME FOR BACK AND NECK

1. Effleurage covering back four times.
2. Kneading four times.
3. Ironing four times.
4. Wringing and picking up four times.
5. Finger kneading and frictions down sides of spine and round scapulae twice.
6. Skin rolling once.
7. Hacking and clapping (percussion) four times.
8. Effleurage four times.

Time taken for back and neck about ten to fifteen minutes.

PROGRAMME FOR BUTTOCKS

1. Effleurage to cover three times.
2. Kneading twice.
3. Reinforced kneading three times.
4. Wringing twice.
5. Percussion (beating, heavy ulnar border hacking) twice.
6. Effleurage three times.

Time taken for buttocks about seven minutes.

N.B. The time taken for the above programmes of massage is only applicable as part of a general body massage. When analysed it is obvious that much more time could be spent on any one area but most general body massage treatments last for one hour. The number of times each manipulation is repeated having covered the area thoroughly once, is a helpful guide when first attempting a complete general body massage, with or without a clock. A general massage is usually started with effleurage, followed by the pressure manipulations, and completed by effleurage again.

Detailed Technique for Body Massage

In all cases the description of the massage will relate to the client's right limbs. This will include massaging the neck and chest, the abdomen, the back, and the buttocks from the right side.

The length of time for each detailed section of massage will vary according to the requirements of the client, as will the number of times each manipulation is performed. The rate at which the massage is performed, like the depth, will again vary according to the required effect of the treatment. It is well to bear in mind that massage, if performed for too long, can become tiring and irritating to the client.

Each of the following descriptions will take into consideration that the massage can be used for independent, localized, and complete treatments, to any section or any one muscle of the body at any time, as well as being used as a method to follow for a general body massage.

RIGHT SHOULDER AND ARM

Position of client and therapist. The client can either be settled comfortably in back lying as described in the general body massage with pillow under head and knees, or she can be treated in a sitting position with her back and head comfortably supported with pillows. Her arm must rest well supported on a pillow and the masseuse takes left walk standing (left foot in front of the right). If the client is sitting on a chair then the therapist could sit by her side, with the pillow and the client's arm resting comfortably on her knees. The arm is a difficult and awkward limb to manoeuvre, so it is of particular importance to pay attention to the most comfortable starting position for both the client and therapist. Before commencing the massage the hands should be warmed, washed, dried, and powdered if necessary.

SHOULDER GIRDLE

Effleurage is first given to the shoulder girdle. The movement begins at the back of the shoulder girdle from the cervical vertebrae across trapezius ending with firm pressure in the supraclavicular glands. The left hand performs this stroke and continues from the base of the hairline forwards again, to end firmly in the same glands increasing the pressure with each stroke. The right hand will be supporting the upper arm at the front. Effleurage is given to the front of the shoulder girdle above the pectoral muscles with the fingers and palm of the right hand to the glands, with the left hand now supporting the back of the shoulder and upper arm. This manipulation is repeated with both hands over deltoid from the top of the shoulder itself into the axillary glands, back and front of the joint.

Kneading with large circular movements is now given to the same area, with palm and fingers of hand using deep pressure over trapezius and rather lighter pressure on the anterior aspect of shoulder girdle across the pectoral muscles.

Finger kneadings and deep frictions follow around and deep into the shoulder joint, starting with fingers together on top of the joint and separating from each other into the axilla back and front (posteriorly and anteriorly).

Effleurage completes the massage to this area.

UPPER ARM

Effleurage to the whole arm from the fingertips to the axilla is the first movement. The left hand works on the back of the arm, and the right hand on the front of the limb. Care must be taken to mould the hands quite accurately to the part keeping the contact smooth and continuous. Each hand works alternately. At the end of the effleurage there should be a deliberate pause followed by gentle pressure to empty the lymph fluid into the lymph glands.

Kneading follows to deltoid, triceps, biceps; both hands press the deltoid muscle against the bone in circular kneading, starting at its origin at the apex of the shoulder and working towards its insertion. *See* Plate 11.

Alternate handed kneading can be employed to massage the anterior and posterior sections of this muscle. This *alternate handed circular kneading* glides from the deltoid muscle into the triceps at the back of the arm, and biceps on the front working again from the proximal attachment of the muscles, distally. *Double handed kneading* can be performed working down in the same manner linking up the movements with short smooth strokes. Great care is essential to massage triceps on the back of the upper arm, as massaging the subcutaneous area of the humerus is most painful, but a very common fault in this area.

Petrissage consisting of *picking up* and *wringing*, using one hand at a time for picking up on each of the above three muscles, is as follows (Plate 12). Starting again with deltoid, the muscle is grasped firmly near its origin with the right hand. The thumb is widely abducted and deltoid is lifted away from and squeezed against the bone in a digging-like manner. Again care with single handed picking up must be taken so as not to pinch and press the fingers and thumb too deeply into the bone whilst manipulating the tissues (Plate 13). The right hand is used on biceps, grasping its bulk medially, beginning from its origin, and lifting the tissues away from the bone and relaxing them, whilst the left hand supports the back of the limb. Single handed picking up follows on triceps with the left hand and when this manipulation is completed, it smoothly changes into *wringing* of deltoid, biceps, and triceps in the same order as before starting from origin towards insertion. The beauty therapist is now working transversely across the length of the muscle fibres, and so, at the same time as changing smoothly into wringing, she now swivels into stride standing. Her feet should be pointing in the same direction that the hands are working. Wringing involves grasping the tissues and firmly lifting them away from the bone, gently twisting the flesh before moving onto another part in one long continuous wave-like flow.

Hacking over deltoid, biceps and triceps follows, but it often proves to be a difficult manipulation to perfect in this area without much perseverance and practice.

Divergent hacking over deltoid starts with both hands close together at the insertion of the muscle, then fanning them out in the direction of its anterior and posterior sections, working up and down its length. The arm is then outwardly rotated, with the elbow bent and still well supported, for hacking transversely across the biceps. If the arm is then medially rotated with an extended elbow, triceps will be easily approached.

Effleurage to the whole arm as before completes the upper arm and shoulder massage. Cover this area with a towel if required.

ELBOW JOINT

Frictions and finger kneadings are given into and around the elbow joint. To penetrate into the back of the joint the forearm should be semi-flexed and pronated. Opening up the front of the elbow joint requires that it should be supinated and extended.

The padded palmar surfaces of the fingertips of the left hand should be used on the back, and of the right hand on and around the front of the joint. Each stationary hand supports the client's wrist and hand alternately.

FOREARM

Effleurage to the whole arm can be performed, if desired, after massage to the elbow joint, but, as there are no lymph glands in this region of importance, an introductory manipulation of stroking from the fingertips to the elbow joint can link up the next manipulation to the muscles of the forearm from the elbow.

Alternate handed kneading of the extensor and flexor group of muscles of the forearm is next given from the elbow towards the wrist. The arm is pronated.

Single handed picking up is given to the same two muscle groups (Plate 14). The left hand picks up the extensor group whilst the right hand holds the forearm in supination and slight flexion. When this movement is completed the left hand glides into supporting the client's wrist and fingers, whilst the right hand in a gliding stroke commences to pick up the flexor group, again from its origin to insertion.

Finger kneadings are performed on the anterior and posterior aspects of the forearm. Both hands can work together if preferred, starting with the pronated extensor group of muscles, working from the origin down towards the wrist between the radius and ulna, stimulating the circulation to the interosseus ligaments and membranes. The forearm is then supinated and the manipulation begins again just below the elbow towards the bulky flexor origin ending between the radius and ulna at the wrist on the anterior aspect of the forearm.

Hacking of both groups follows and the client's co-operation in pronating and supinating the forearm will be required to sustain continuous and effective percussion.

WRIST JOINT

Finger kneading and deep frictions are given to back and front of the wrist joint. When working on the posterior aspect the wrist should be flexed, but should be extended when frictioning the anterior aspect so that deep penetration into the joint occurs.

HAND AND FINGERS

Deep palmar and dorsal kneading between the two hands is first applied from the wrist to the fingertips.

Thumb kneading with the right and left hands follows to the thenar and hypothenar eminences of the thumb and little finger (Plate 15). Care is taken here to massage into the crevices and spaces of the bones and into the interosseus ligaments and intrinsic muscles of the palm of the hand. Both its anterior and posterior aspect should be covered.

Wringing and picking up can be applied to the fleshy ball of thumb and little finger, but the technique is adapted by using the masseuse's index finger and thumb of both hands in a delicate but nonetheless deep manipulation lifting the muscles away from the bone and squeezing from side to side. *See* Plate 16.

Stroking to the fingers follows from the tips to the roots, usually pairing the ring and index finger, middle and little finger together. The thumb is treated separately, but care must be taken to cover all aspects of the phalanges.

Spiral finger kneadings are given with the fingers and thumbs of one hand, whilst the other supports the base of the client's palm. The movement consists of small corkscrew-like kneadings round the fingers from tip to root, maintaining firm contact, and it produces a pleasant warm sensory feeling, but special care should be taken around the joints. *Stroking* finishes the massage to the hand.

Hacking to the whole arm can now be applied. The therapist should stride stand at about the level of the elbow, parallel with the upper arm. With the forearm pronated she works transversely from the wrist upwards, fingers striking across the forearm to the elbow. Swivelling into walk standing, the fingers turn round the elbow onto the back of the upper arm where triceps is hacked upwards towards its insertion. The operator then swivels into stride standing again, hacking across deltoid over the biceps, asking the client to supinate the slightly flexed forearm. She then hacks down biceps lightly across the front of the elbow and down the medial side of the forearm to the wrist.

Effleurage to the whole limb completes the massage to the arm.

N.B. Stroking is a manipulation which should be utilized as a link manipulation whenever possible to maintain continuity between all movements. It can follow the normal paths of effleurage without ending in lymph glands to act merely as a connector, or it can be used as a soothing and relaxing, or stimulating manipulation.

RIGHT LEG

Position. If the leg is to be massaged as part of a general body massage, the client would be most comfortable in back lying with an extra pillow behind her head and another pillow which will be used in varying ways to support the leg whilst massaging it. Alternatively she can be comfortably settled in long sitting if the treatment is confined to her limbs only. The beauty therapist must consider her stance most carefully when treating the lower limb. This applies to the back also. Body weight in both cases is essential for a thorough and effective treatment. Left walk standing is the most convenient position, swinging into stride standing when the manipulations change direction.

Full support of the heavy lower limb demands frequent changing of pillow position. The combination of the therapist's position and correct limb support requires much practice to be perfected, so that the rhythm and continuity of the massage is unaffected. It is easier to treat a leg standing, but if the plinth or couch is too low the sitting position has to be adopted to prevent strain on the therapist's back.

Once the client is comfortable, warm, and relaxed, and the therapist's hands are washed and clean, the massage begins. The leg to be treated should be resting on a pillow in relaxed outward rotation, with the hip and knee slightly flexed, and with the foot and ankle free.

The therapist stands in the left walk position at about the level of the ankle joint.

Effleurage, starting with the hands on the inner and outer sides of the foot and using body weight over the thigh, ends in the lymph glands in the groin (femoral triangle); this stroke should cover the anterior surface of the limb. The second stroke will cover the medial and lateral sides of the leg, the left hand being taken high up onto the gluteal mass laterally and returning into the groin. The third stroke must cover the posterior aspect of the limb surfacing to the front of the thigh, at the top of the leg, curving into the groin, and with slight pressure emphasis on the lymph glands at the end of the stroke.

Circular kneading, beginning with the left hand high on the gluteal mass, follows. The right hand rests on the adductor group of muscles and, when the two hands are level, alternate handed kneading continues down towards the knee. Care is taken not to massage into the femoral triangle for obvious reasons. Kneading of the anterior and posterior aspect of the thigh follows. The left hand changes onto the quadriceps muscles and the right slides to the back of the thigh onto the hamstrings (Plate 17). The left hand again starts the manipulation high up near to the quadriceps origin and, when level, works in conjunction with the right hand down towards the knee. The position of stride standing is adopted, and picking up is given to the adductors and quadriceps starting at the origins of the muscle groups working towards their insertions. *Double handed picking up* of rectus femoris can be applied, again from its pelvic origin down towards its insertion, and this can be followed by *wringing* to the thigh in the same way and pattern.

Hacking and clapping of these muscles is given followed by effleurage as before; the thigh is covered.

Plate 1.   Effleurage into the femoral triangle

Plate 2.   Effleurage into the axillae

Plate 3.   Effleurage to the back

Plate 4.   Finger kneading

Plate 5.   Ironing

Plate 6. Wringing

Plate 7. Skin rolling

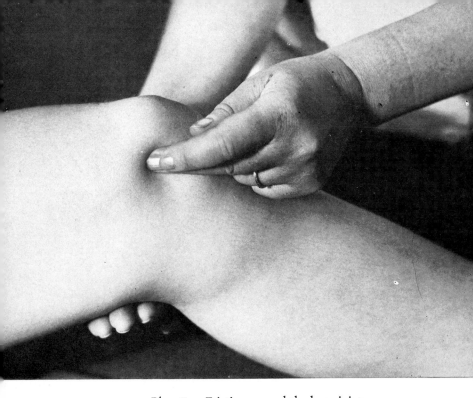

Plate 8.   Frictions round the knee joint

Plate 9.   Hacking

Plate 10.   Clapping

Plate 11.   Kneading the biceps

Plate 12.   Wringing the triceps

Plate 13.   Single handed picking up of the biceps

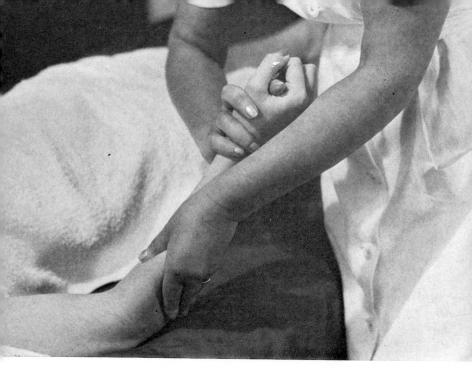

Plate 14.   Single handed picking up of the forearm extensor muscles

Plate 15.   Thumb kneading to the hand

Plate 16.   Wringing the hypothenar eminence

Plate 17.   Kneading the quadriceps and the hamstrings

Plate 18.   Alternate handed kneading above and below the knee joint

Plate 19.   Wringing the calf muscles

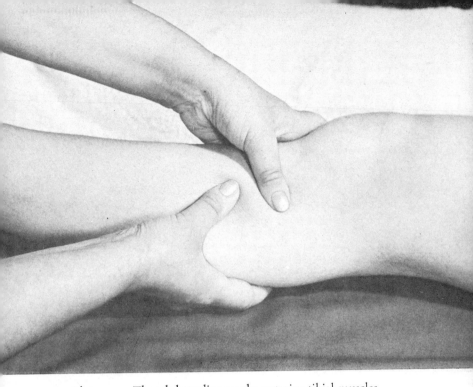

Plate 20. Thumb kneading to the anterior tibial muscles

Plate 21. Stroking the foot

Plate 22.   Double handed picking up of the neck

Plate 23.   Divergent hacking over the scapular muscles

Plate 24.   Effleurage to the supra-clavicular glands

Plate 25.   Picking up on the back

Plate 26.   Transverse clapping
Plate 27.   Beating the buttocks

Plate 28.　　Alternate method of stroking the neck and chest

Plate 29.　　Kneading of the small intestine

Plate 30.   Stroking the ascending and transverse colon

Plate 31.   Kneading the abdominal wall

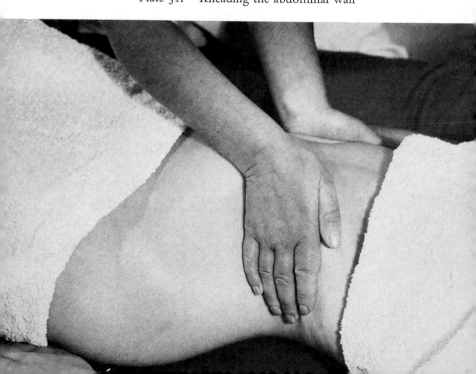

KNEE JOINT

Position. Walk stride position is adopted and effleurage with both hands is given around the knee joint finishing in the popliteal lymph glands at the back of the knee.

Alternate handed kneading is given to the knee above and below and either side, paying particular attention to the patella (Plate 18).

Finger kneading and frictions round the patella, into the joint round the condyles, and at the back of the joint, are followed by movements of the patella up and down and from side to side.

N.B. When massaging above and below the joint with kneading change foot position to stride standing, place one hand above the patella and the other below, squeezing the tissues towards each hand in a digging-like manner. This is most effective on the deep structures of the joint.

Effleurage completes the massage.

LOWER LEG

Position. The beauty therapist is in walk standing position. The pillow is placed under the client's thigh, leaving the lower leg free, flexed, and relaxed.

Effleurage, in the same manner as for the thigh, ends here in the popliteal lymph glands and the back of the knee.

Kneading to the posterior calf muscles with the right hand, and the anterior tibial muscles with the left follows.

Picking up and wringing to the calf muscles (Plate 19) whilst smoothly changing into stride standing is next.

Single handed picking up to the calf muscles can be given with the right hand, whilst the left supports the knee. Once again the operator changes into walk standing whilst thumb and finger kneadings are performed round the head of the fibula and anterior tibial muscles towards the ankle (Plate 20). Care must be taken to avoid the sharp anterior border of the tibia, or shin bone.

Light hacking with the leg rolled inwards in stride position to the same muscles is followed by *hacking* and *clapping* of the posterior tibial muscles in walk standing position, with the leg now rolled out again.

Effleurage is applied to the whole limb after the pillow has once more been placed under the knee and lower leg, which should then be covered.

ANKLE JOINT AND FOOT

Stroke from the toes to the back of the ankle in walk standing, the right hand on top and the left underneath the foot (Plate 21).

Finger knead the Achilles tendon and round the crevices of the ankle joint.

Knead the anterior and posterior aspect of the foot between the two hands, deep kneading into the sole of the foot starting from the ankle.

Thumb knead the dorsum of the foot and the lateral border, starting behind the heel working towards the roots of the toes.

Stroke and spiral finger knead each toe from tip to root.

General hacking and clapping to the whole leg is followed by *effleurage* to the whole of the lower limb.

BACK MASSAGE

For the purposes of detailed description below the back will be divided. In the programme for a general massage, it will be seen that these two areas have been combined into one whole area, that is, back, neck, and shoulders.

UPPER BACK AND NECK

Position. The client should be in prone lying with one pillow under her abdomen and another under the front of the ankles. Her forehead rests on the back of her hands with elbows bent or, if she is comfortable and can turn her head sideways, with the arms slightly bent but tucked down by her sides. The beauty therapist stands in left walk standing on the left side of the client but should be able to massage the back from either side. Only the area to be treated should be uncovered.

Effleurage starts with both hands placed at the base of the occiput and hair-line. They are drawn firmly down the neck and divide one to each side over the upper borders of trapezius to end firmly in the supra-clavicular glands. The next stroke of effleurage commences from the medial borders of the scapula and thoracic vertebrae and each hand fans out over the scapula across trapezius into the corresponding axilla.

Finger kneading either side of the cervical spine down the lateral side of the neck and across the upper border of trapezius follow. Careful attention is paid to the supra- and infra-spinatus muscles. This area is bony, and too much pressure can cause discomfort.

Double handed picking up of the neck follows (first to seventh cervical vertebrae) from the root of the hair downwards to the upper borders of trapezius, where the hands separate picking up independently, but with the pressure working towards each other over the upper borders of trapezius as the tissues are lifted and squeezed. *See* Plate 22.

Wringing is next, from the scalp downwards, covering the whole of this area across the scapulae and neck.

Frictions down either side of the spine, into trapezius erector spine and around the bony edges of the scapulae, are followed by *hacking.*

Divergent hacking over the scapular muscles and across the upper borders of trapezius can be performed still in walk standing (Plate 23). Or as in wringing the therapist can swivel into stride standing and hack the whole area transversely across.

Effleurage as before completes the work in this area.

LOWER BACK, NECK, AND SHOULDER MASSAGE

Position. The client is prone lying with pillow under abdomen and ankles. The back is uncovered from the iliac crests upwards.

The beauty therapist stands in the walk position using the body weight.

Effleurage with both hands from the iliac crests either side of the spine to the supra-clavicular glands is the first stroke (Plate 24). Each succeeding stroke begins at the iliac crest but nearer towards the lateral side of the back, and ends in the axilla until the whole of this area is covered. This usually takes three strokes. Firm pressure is used on the upward stroke, only light contact being maintained on the return journey with the fingertips, to start to effleurage again.

Circular kneading. The hands work on either side of the spine with deep pressure, either alternately or both together. The same order as effleurage is followed to cover the back, but the manipulations all begin at the top of the back, either side of the neck working downwards to the pelvis.

Ironing is the next manipulation. Swivel into stride standing. Place the left hand reinforced with the right hand near the axilla on the right side of the trunk. Iron with slightly flexed elbows so directing deep pressure against the bone. Work downwards towards the iliac crests, then up again and across the top of the shoulders, back down, and up, until the whole area has been completely covered. It will be found that there is some difficulty in treating the side of the body nearest to the operator and so the hands can be turned either up or down to overcome this problem. Gentle rotation from the hips and ankles can help to obtain deep pressure and rhythm, emphasizing the use of body weight.

Picking up and wringing are excluded in a general massage of the back if it is too thin and bony as the back muscles are flat and thin. However, on most backs there is usually sufficient adipose tissue to enable these manipulations to be performed most comfortably (Plate 25). This stage of the general body massage is very often the most relaxing and pleasing part of the whole massage for the client. If the technique of these petrissage manipulations is well executed the client may drift into a light sleep. The same stance and order of work as for ironing is adopted for wringing and picking up, covering the whole back smoothly and methodically without any breaks between one manipulation or the other. Body weight again is used and emphasis is placed on rhythm according to the manipulation.

Finger kneading and frictions follow but the position of stride standing is once again changed to that of left walk standing. Kneading and frictions begin from the base of the skull and hairline down either side of the spine of the vertebrae. Deep pressure is essential here to be effective on the erector spinae muscles which lie mainly between the transverse processes and the spine of the vertebrae. Also the joints and ligaments of the spine will be benefited. Care is taken to avoid pressure on the bony joints but to massage deeply round them, and round the borders and spine of the scapulae. Here and across the upper borders of the trapezii trigger spots of muscle tension may be found, so care must be taken not to cause discomfort.

Skin rolling transversely across the back is performed in stride standing. Starting at the axilla, roll the tissues in over the shoulders towards the spine. Move inch by inch smoothly down the back until one side has been completely covered. The side of the back furthest away from the operator poses a little difficulty and the tissues on this side are rolled by the thumbs from the spine towards the lateral side of the back, to the mid-axillary line, but again starting across the top of the shoulder girdle.

Percussion. The client slightly flexes her neck, supporting it on the pillow or hands. *Longitudinal light hacking* down the cervical vertebrae changes into heavier hacking down the thoracic and lumbar regions with the therapist positioned in walk standing. Still in the same position divergent hacking starts with hands together in the cervical region fanning them outwards across the muscles. The hacking continues down the length of the back, bringing each stroke into the centre of the spine to diverge again. Stride walk position is adapted for transverse hacking and clapping (Plate 26), which starts at the right axilla, and works down and up the back, until it has all been covered on either side of the spine.

Effleurage concludes the back massage and the area is covered.

BUTTOCKS AND GLUTEAL MASSAGE

Position of the client remains unchanged. The therapist takes walk standing position, and uncovers the area from the waist down to the top of the thigh.

Effleurage, from mid-line over the lumbar region with both hands outwards towards the groin, starts the massage. The following strokes become lower until the gluteal fold is reached.

Alternate circular kneading follows with one hand on each gluteal mass again from mid-line outwards.

Ironing each side separately can be given.

Wringing and picking up in this area may only be possible on the top of the hips and into the waist because of the density of these heavy tissues.

Finger kneading and frictions can be applied around the sacrum and deep into all the joints of this area.

Hacking, beating, and pounding are given with the operator in stride standing and if desired over a towel to prevent any discomfort (Plate 27).

Effleurage completes the massage.

NECK AND CHEST

Position of the client can be in back lying or sitting up, depending on whether the massage is included as part of a general body massage, when a minimum of movement is essential. Support behind the head with pillows ensures that the neck and chest muscles are relaxed. One pillow placed under the knees takes the strain off the abdominal muscles. The therapist is in walk standing position on the right of the client. The arms should be relaxed and the area to be treated uncovered.

Effleurage down the lateral sides of the neck into the supraclavicular glands is the first stroke. The next stroke following the same path down the side of the neck with each hand fans outwards across the pectoral muscles into the axilla. An alternate method of stroking or effleurage (Plate 28) is to place the left hand on the lateral left side of the client's neck, drawing it smoothly downwards across the left sterno-mastoid muscle, over the sternum and right pectoral muscles, into the right axilla. The right hand then follows the same path, starting on the client's right side and ending in the left axilla. Another stroke, using both hands together across the front of the chest and pectoral muscles, is to place the left hand at the fold of the left axilla and the right hand on the right fold, taking both hands across the chest and pectorals at the same time to the opposite axilla.

Finger kneading down the lateral sides of the neck and upper border of trapezius from origin to insertion follows. The sterno-mastoid muscle is finger kneaded. Care must be taken not to encroach on the front of the throat as this is most unpleasant for the client.

Light palmar kneading, if the area permits, across the pectoral muscles and chest is next, followed again by *finger kneading* round the clavicle and sternum and over platysma.

The breast tissue must not be encroached upon in this area.

Light divergent hacking and vibrations across the pectoral muscles, followed by *effleurage* as before, completes this massage.

Abdominal Massage

An abdominal massage is often requested as a special treatment, and up to half an hour can be spent massaging the abdominal wall and the abdominal organs in order to promote digestion. However, although there are schools of thought that believe this massage serves little purpose, many people still prefer this old-fashioned method of treatment to other forms, and those who are dieting or fasting in an effort to lose weight find it invaluable and particularly useful. Therefore the beauty therapist should have a good knowledge of the digestive tract and the detailed abdominal massage in case she is requested to give one. It would constitute a complete treatment in its own right and should never be hurried, nor included in a general massage of the body.

However, when an abdominal massage is included in the general programme, it is only the muscular abdominal wall which is treated; weight-conscious clients welcome this part of the massage.

Position. The client should be placed so that all strain and tension is taken off the abdominal muscles. If she is in back lying the knees must be flexed and well supported. An alternate position could be to raise the back of the couch and support her leaning backwards against pillows. She should be well covered with only the abdomen exposed and her arms relaxed by the sides of her body. It is essential that she is as relaxed as possible, and deep breathing exercises can be practised, or shown her, before the treatment commences. An abdominal massage should not be attempted until at least one hour after a meal, and the bladder should be empty otherwise it is uncomfortable.

If possible a rest of twenty minutes is advocated after the massage has been completed. Scars on the abdomen should be noted and enquired about, and gentle palpation will indicate if there is any abnormal tenderness that would contra-indicate a massage in this region. Bony points in this area must be particularly noted, for excruciating pain can be caused through careless technique. The iliac crests and lower borders of the ribs are the main areas where dragging of the tissues causes discomfort. It is of the utmost importance in this area to ensure that one manipulation glides smoothly and rhythmically into the other ensuring continuity of work throughout the whole massage. A detailed abdominal massage may build up in time from ten to forty minutes if required. The aim of an abdominal massage is to perfect digestion and absorption by promoting a better blood supply to the organs, so improving their nutrition and stimulating the cells to provide a richer flow of digestive juices. The involuntary muscle action is simulated and intestinal stasis prevented. These movements help to mix the food with the juices and push it along the different parts of the tract. When massaging the abdominal wall it is well to bear in mind its function, which is to help to empty the contents of the digestive tract, and also to support and hold in place the abdominal organs. Other effects of massage on the abdominal organs can be found in Chapter 4.

The therapist should have warm dry hands and always stand on the right side of the client, starting in the left walk position. During the abdominal massage care should be taken when working with one hand only to support the client with the other hand, and not to use it to support the therapist on the couch, or on the client.

PROGRAMME AND ORDER OF WORK

1. Stroking of abdominal wall (muscles and fat).
2. Stomach.
3. Liver.
4. Small intestine (Plate 29).
5. Colon (ascending, transverse, and descending) (Plate 30).
6. Abdominal wall (detailed massage).

ABDOMINAL WALL

Stroking from the back of the waist forwards and obliquely downwards towards the groin introduces the abdominal massage. It can be performed either with one hand following the other covering the whole abdominal wall, or with both hands on either side working together. This accustoms the client to the therapist's touch, helping to promote complete relaxation which is so essential in this massage. *See* Plate 31.

STOMACH

Stroking in stride standing is first given from the left lateral side of the stomach forwards to its exit into the duodenum at the pyloric sphincter. Each hand works alternately giving firmer pressure with every new stroke. Care must be taken not to drag the tissues across the iliac crest and not to lean on the abdomen with the forearms at any stage in this massage. This is a common fault easily made.

Kneading using the right hand consists of a squeezing and relaxing manipulation lifting the ulnar border of the hand under the lower ribs as though trying to cup the stomach in the hand itself. This starts from the left side of the waist and works forwards to the pylorus.

Stroking as before completes the stomach massage.

LIVER

The client turns a little to her left side.

Stroking begins from the back over the area of the liver and works forwards with alternate hands. The pressure should be firm and deep as the liver is protected by the ribs.

Kneading follows. Place the left hand over the back of the area of the liver and the right hand over its anterior surface, on the front of the lower ribs. The kneading should be slow and deep, each hand working alternately, cupping the lower border of the liver upwards with the ulnar side of the right hand.

Percussion, consisting of stimulating hacking, is given over the whole area of the liver.

Stroking as before completes the massage.

SMALL INTESTINE

Kneading in stride standing is first given. The kneading over the small intestine is modified to the shape of the structures to be stimulated in the following way. The two hands are placed transversely across the abdomen. The tissues are moved with a gentle pushing movement from the padded heels of the hands on the right side of the navel towards the fingertips on the left side. They are then pulled back in reverse to the heels of the hands. The procedure begins again. This movement almost resembles the swell of a wave on the sea. It is thought to cause a manipulation of the intestine lying underneath between the fingers and the heels of the hands, and in this way massages it and simulates its movement. This transverse kneading slides into a form of kneading, moving the structures round the navel, first one way, and then back the other way in a clockwise and anti-clockwise direction. The heel of the left hand works towards the fingers of the right. In this way, working round the abdomen, the whole of the intestine may be mechanically stimulated. The hands then glide obliquely across the abdomen and the tissues are squeezed and relaxed between them, the fingers and ulnar border of one hand working with the heels of the other.

Vibrations using either the right hand by itself or reinforced with the left, move transversely across the abdomen from the left side of the abdominal wall to the right, working back to the beginning and repeating the movement several times across the abdomen over the whole area of the intestine.

COLON

Stroking, again following the direction of the flow of the contents of the digestive tract, begins from the right side of the pelvis and travels up over the area of the ascending, across the transverse, and down the area of the descending colon.

Different methods of stroking are employed here and it entirely depends upon the therapist which method is adopted. One technique is to stand in stride standing and place the left hand pointing to the groin over the area of the ascending colon drawing it upwards towards, and deeply into, the right side of the waist. Now the left hand is turned and stroked across the area of the transverse colon, turning it again at the left side to stroke downwards along the path of the descending colon. The right hand firmly traces the same path the left hand has travelled, ending over the descending colon in the left pelvic area with firm pressure.

This stroking of the colon should be repeated several times with gently increasing pressure along its course.

Kneading follows. Because of the situation and shape of the structures being treated the hypothenar eminence of the right hand is used to knead the ascending colon. The therapist stands in left walk standing and starts from the right-hand side of the pelvis working up over the ascending colon into the waist. The kneading should be fairly deep. At the waist the beauty therapist swivels into stride standing and kneads across the transverse colon with the palmar surface of her hand. At the left side she once again turns into left walk standing and at the same time continues to knead deeply downwards over the area of the descending colon towards the left groin, with the thenar eminence of the right hand. This enables her to cup the kneading into the iliac fossa without dragging the tissues across the bony iliac crest.

Vibrations, either with the fingertips or the whole hand, follow the same course as the other manipulations over the area of the colon.

Stroking as before to the colon completes the massage of this organ.

ABDOMINAL WALL

This massage to the abdominal wall can either be done at the beginning or at the end of a detailed abdominal massage, but not in the middle of the massage of the organs.

Stroking is the first manipulation to be performed. The therapist is in the left walk position and, placing her hands on either side of the waist well to the back, draws them firmly down to the groin. The stroking can be performed with one hand at a time or both hands together covering the whole of the abdominal wall in three strokes. Transverse stroking from the left side of the waist and lower ribs towards the right side with alternate hands over the transverse muscle, and oblique stroking from one side of the abdomen and lower ribs to the opposite groin following the direction of the oblique muscles, is another method of stroking the muscular abdominal wall.

Kneading follows in walk standing with the left and right hands placed on either side of the lower ribs, briskly working towards the middle and downwards to the pubis.

Wringing and picking up deep into the waist over the lower ribs, and if possible over the anterior wall of the abdomen, follows. If the client is well endowed with adipose tissue, and has poor muscle tone, wringing and picking up will be most beneficial on the anterior wall of the abdomen; otherwise it is confined to the lateral sides, at the tops of the hips and waist regions, where there is more fat and protection from underlying bone.

Light hacking, changing into stride standing, across the whole of the abdominal wall starting from the left side working up and down towards the right, is the last manipulation.

Stroking as before completes the abdominal wall massage.

Modification of Treatments

SPECIAL POINTS TO BE CONSIDERED

OBESITY

In cases of obesity the work required will have to be vigorous, heavy, and deep. Skin rolling may well replace kneading, especially round the great trochanter on the thigh and around the medial condyles of the femora. Where the upper arm is obese care should be taken when employing skin rolling because it can be most uncomfortable and result in a burning sensation. Skin rolling may be performed over the lower ribs and around the waist in such cases but is completely contra-indicated over the anterior wall of the abdomen under all circumstances, as there is no bone to protect the underlying organs or against which to roll the fatty tissues.

Breast massage for any condition is not performed in beauty therapy. Skin rolling may be used for obese clients over the gluteal muscles but generally speaking, even in extremely fatty clients, the tissues here are too dense to put this manipulation into practice. Wringing, picking up, hacking and clapping, beating and pounding can be applied where there is much adipose tissue. All the manipulations should be brisk and deep.

RELAXATION

When a client requires a treatment purely for relaxation all stimulating manipulations should be avoided. Emphasis is placed

on the back massage. The manipulations should be monotonously
slow and rhythmic. Ironing and kneading prove to be the most
relaxing and soothing; stroking replaces effleurage. This takes the
form of long slow strokes from the occiput to the sacrum with
the touch firm but light and gentle.

STIMULATION

For a client who lacks energy and feels debilitated a brisk stimulating massage would incorporate light manipulations with the
accent on percussion, petrissage (wringing, picking up, and skin
rolling), and brisk stroking. They would be carried out at a fairly
quick but even rhythm. Deep vibrations and hacking performed
down the vertebrae over the exit of the spinal nerves are said to
stimulate the central nervous system and the effect should leave
the client feeling refreshed, alive, and invigorated. Local vibrations and hacking performed with the fingertips over the peripheral nerves will produce a similar effect.

GENERAL ACHES AND PAINS

Providing there is no medical condition the relief of rheumaticky
aches and pains, knots of tension, or accumulated fatigue products
can be effected by deep massage. Frictions into thickened
structures and around joints down the long back muscles can be
performed. Deep petrissage and ironing of muscle groups interspersed with plenty of effleurage will prove to be most beneficial.
Usually the client herself indicates the whereabouts of her
particular ache of the day and the therapist can concentrate on
this area, incorporating the appropriate manipulations, with deep
pressure requiring much use of body weight.

OVERTONED AND CONTRACTED MUSCLES

Percussion is completely omitted.

Requires careful slow rhythmic kneading and petrissage.
Stroking would replace effleurage. This can be most effective
over the pectoral muscles, for example, where percussion would
be contra-indicated if the client were round-shouldered and the

pectorals contracted and shortened. In cases of muscular cramp where the muscles go into spasm, deep slow kneading helps to relax and stretch out the spasm. A shortened tendo-achilles or tight hamstrings would benefit by the above treatment, including finger kneadings, providing it were deep and slow, discouraging further contraction. Bulky well-toned muscles would require a relaxing massage without any percussion.

SLACK AND FLABBY MUSCLES

Untoned muscles which are slack and flabby and have lost their elasticity can be nourished and stimulated with brisk massage. Usually it is the aging processes of the body, as well as the kind of life led, which contribute to the sagging muscles and skin. Drastic dieting and weight loss is another contributory factor. Finger kneadings, vibrations, and light hacking in the region of platysma over the neck and chest will help to provide this area with the tonic effect if may need. Brisk kneadings, clapping, and hacking are used over the other areas where the tissues have lost tone and where nourishment and stimulation are the first consideration. Later on, petrissage can be incorporated into the treatment, as the tone improves and further stimulation is required without fear of over-stretching the skin.

OEDEMA

Too much standing and drinking cups of tea can lead to gravitational oedema. The ankles and feet are puffy and possibly the hands may appear swollen too. Under these circumstances the client can be given a special massage to help the lymph carry away the retention of fluid. The arms would be supported with pillows above the level of the axillae and the legs would be raised above the groin. Squeezing kneading, starting from the proximal end of the limb combined with effleurage, would proceeed down its length, section by section, working up over the massaged segments again each time a new area is squeezed. The hands squeeze the tissues together until the whole limb has been covered slowly and methodically, interspersing effleurage at every stage. There would be no doubt at all in the therapist's mind if a medical condition were present due to varying causes. The area would pit leaving finger marks if medical attention was indicated. These would fill with fluid again, and the skin would be pale and cool. Sometimes the face, legs, and hands swell before menstruating and many doctors prescribe a diuretic at this time, to rid tissues of excess fluid. Water retention, over-weight, and 'it's my glands' often go hand in hand with obesity, but abnormal water retention in the body could lead to the abdomen, hips, and thighs being grossly distended. This is easily distinguishable from the normal fatty layers, for the skin is shiny, the navel protrudes, and there would be a rippling of the tissue fluids as the client moves, across the abdomen and thighs. Where there is any doubt ask the client to consult her doctor.

Head and Scalp Massage

Position. The client can either sit on a chair in a forward leaning position with the forehead and arms resting comfortably on several pillows supported on a table, or she can be treated in prone lying with the forehead resting on the back of the hands in a forward position. The massage is given in walk standing with the hands on either side of the head.

Stroking starting from the brow with the fingertips to the base of the occiput is first given. The fingers are drawn slowly through the hair several times with slight pressure on the scalp.

Finger kneadings are next applied, again working from the hair-line of the brow to the base of the occiput; care must be taken to move the scalp on the skull for full effect and to deepen the pressure over any areas of tension.

Running vibrations starting from the brow and vibrating to the base of the occiput through the hair are next given, with the hands on either side of the head, as in the previous manipulations.

Stroking as before completes this massage.

Face Massage

Position. The client can be in back lying with the head supported by pillows or sitting in a backward reclining position again well supported. The therapist stands or sits behind the client.

Stroking with both hands diverging from the centre of the brow to the sides of the temple in front of the ear begins this delicate but firm massage. The next strokes are given with padded surfaces of the thumbs. Starting from the bridge of the nose over the cheek bones with a lifting movement towards the ear; from the upper lip outwards towards the ear, continuing above the chin still accenting the pressure in an upwards direction over the lower cheek, again towards the ear; with the last stroke being performed by the pads of the fingers from under the chin, throat, and jaw to the ear.

Finger kneading midline to the forehead to the ears follows. This is performed with the pads of either the middle or the index fingers working on all the small muscles of the face from midline outwards and upwards, towards the ear. Special attention must be paid to finger knead into the tempero-mandibular joint in front of the ear.

Point hacking is an adaptation of hacking because of the delicacy of the facial structures. It consists of light hacking using the padded parts of the fifth, fourth, and third fingers in a tapping-like manner and is given over the brow, cheeks, and chin lifting the tissues upwards.

Vibrations either with the fingertips or flat hand can be given over the same areas, and especially over the exit of the facial nerve in front of the mastoid process.

Stroking as before completes the massage.

SPECIAL POINTS TO BE CONSIDERED

EYES

The eyes should be closed throughout the massage and the following massage incorporated into the general facial massage.

Stroking, starting at the outside corner of the eyes, continues lightly over the lids with the pads of the thumb or index fingers to the inner corner.

Finger kneading, superficial and delicate, follows in the same manner to the upper lids, with the tip of the index finger.

Stroking follows as before.

Stroking continues around the eyes starting this time from the inner corner below the eyes and finishing at the inner corner above in a circular direction.

Finger kneading follows in the same direction around the orbicularis occuli muscle.

Stroking in a circular direction as before completes this massage.

MOUTH

Particular attention must be paid to the area around the mouth, care being taken to lift the corners of the mouth when applying all the manipulations.

TIME

Time for both the head and face can last between twenty and thirty minutes each.

Modification of Treatment for Head and Face

SPECIAL POINTS TO BE CONSIDERED

RELAXATION

If a client has difficulty in relaxing, a head and facial massage can be most beneficial, especially as tension very often shows in the face. All percussion would be omitted; frictions and finger kneadings to the scalp would be emphasized. Double handed picking up could be incorporated in the head massage to the 'scruff' of the neck rhythmically and slowly. Gentle stroking from mid-jawline encroaching outwards across the shoulders can be included in the facial massage, whilst the finger kneadings from the jawline can continue round the back of the neck along the base of the hair-line, upper borders of trapezius, and into the sterno-mastoid muscle from origin to insertion.

SLACK SKIN AND MUSCLES

In the area of throat, face, and neck, these require stimulating brisk manipulations lifting but not stretching the tissues further. Tapping under the chin or point hacking will have a tonic effect. Cream or oil could be used in conjunction with a facial massage. (*See Care of the Skin* by the same author, Heinemann, 1975.)

N.B. Whenever a tonic effect on muscles is required in the body, or a weight loss is desired, it would be advisable for the client to practise a scheme of active exercises and to follow a suitable diet, for the massage to be fully effective.

Modifications for Stiffness in the Joints

Providing that the beauty therapist knows why the joint is stiff and that no medical condition exists, the following modifications can be incorporated into a general body massage. If the cause of stiffness is in doubt the advice of a doctor should be sought before massage is given.

SHOULDER JOINT

Massage should be vigorous to all the muscles which act on the joint. This includes the shoulder, arm, neck, chest, and back, and the whole shoulder girdle. Deep frictions and finger kneadings are applied to the joint itself followed by plenty of effleurage and hacking. Passive movements should be given followed by mobilizing exercises of the quick swinging variety.

ELBOW JOINT

Massage to the whole arm, particularly the muscles above and below the joint. Frictions as above are applied to the joint structures followed by passive and active movements.

WRIST, HAND, AND FINGER JOINTS

Massage to the whole arm is given but with emphasis on the forearm and hand. Special consideration and care is taken around the wrist and small joints of the hand with frictions and finger kneadings. Passive movements and exercises particularly for mobility are stressed.

BACK AND SPINE JOINTS

Massage should be deep and vigorous. Double handed picking up to the back of the neck can be given, followed by deep finger kneadings and frictions to the joints of the spine, sterno-mastoid, and into the erector spinae muscles. In the lumbar and sacral regions ironing can replace wringing and picking up, which is found to be most comforting.

HIP JOINT

Massage with the client lying on her side with a pillow placed between her knees for comfort enables the therapist to massage the hip adequately. Particular attention is paid to the gluteal and thigh muscles and also those of the lumbar region. Passive movements followed by mobilizing exercises should be given.

KNEE JOINT

Massage to the whole leg is given, particular attention being paid to quadriceps. Deep frictions around the knee joint and patella with the knee in semi-flexion should be followed again by passive movements, patella movements, and active exercises.

ANKLE, FOOT, AND TOE JOINTS

Massage is given to the whole leg, including the muscles of the thigh, the anterior tibial muscles, and the muscles of the sole of the foot. Finger kneading and frictions are emphasized down the tibialis anterior muscle, round the crevices of the ankle joint, and into the deep short foot muscles. Passive movements to the ankle and toes should be followed by mobilizing and strengthening exercises. Faradic foot-baths are excellent in stimulating the muscles of the arches of the feet.

SCARS

Massage to scars should consist of manipulations which try to lift the scar tissue from the underlying structures and prevent the muscles from becoming caught up in the healing process. Oil is the best medium to use when massaging scars for it allows a greater stretching of the skin.

HEAT TREATMENTS

Wax, steam, or dry heat treatments, or baths, can be applied to the tissues or joints prior to massage. They can be used to soothe and ease pain, or merely to relax the client, or as a slimming aid.

Modification of massage for men.

In men the skin is thicker, tougher, and hairier. The subcutaneous layer contains little fat and so their tissues are firmer and more resistant. Also the muscles are toned and resilient. A toning massage is required for men in which the invigorating manipulations of wringing, picking up, alternate handed kneading, finger kneading, deep effleurage, and percussion are mainly used. These should be performed with greater depth, using all the body weight, at a more rigorous and faster rhythm than the general massage for woman. A full massage for men is often condensed into half an hour. Here the arms, chest, and light abdominal massage precedes the massage to the back of the legs and back massage, both of which are applied with the client in prone lying. Concentration of massage with wringing and finger kneading around the upper boarders of the trapezius muscle and upper back region relieves tension and tenseness, commonly found in this area. A good vegetable massage oil or an appropriate essential oil will enable the skin to be stretched without tearing, and greater pressure to be applied. Removal of excess oil with hot towels, or an astringent completes the treatment.

6. *Bones*

The study of bones is called osteology. Bones can be likened to the woodwork of a primitive cottage providing the body with its basic shape. This framework of bones is called the skeleton (Figure 1). The skeleton is divided into an axial part consisting of the bones of the head and trunk, and an appendicular part consisting of the bones of the limbs, or extremities (arms and legs).

The structure of bones is that of one kind of connective tissue, in which various calcium salts are laid down in the basic ground substance, so providing the body with one of its hardest and toughest structures. The articulating or joint surfaces are covered in hyaline cartilage, which helps to give ease and smoothness of movement in the joints. Elsewhere the outside covering of bone is called the periosteum. This is a tough membrane which provides a bed for the blood vessels, nerves, and lymphatics to rest in before branching out to feed, nourish, and supply the rest of the bone. If the bone was to be stripped of the periosteum, it would die.

Two kinds of bone are to be found in the body: compact or hard dense bone, and cancellous or spongy bone. The heavy compact bone can be found around the lighter cancellous bone, forming a hard outer layer. Red marrow fills in the centre, or medulla, of the hard bones and where there is no marrow cavity as such, it is found in the space between the cancellous bone. It is mainly in the red marrow found in the cancellous bone tissue that the red blood corpuscles are found. Fat can also be found in the spongy bone tissue, and yellow marrow in the shafts of long bones. The surface of the bones sometimes is heavily ridged, roughened, or bumpy. These different features are due to the pull of the muscles which are attached to the bones.

The function of the bones is to give shape and support to the body. They provide rigid surfaces for the attachment of muscles, ligaments, and fascia. The bones provide the muscles with flexible levers moving at the joints which connect them up. Usually the more fixed bone is the point from which the muscle originates, and the moving bone is its insertion point. Protection is given by the skeleton to underlying organs and structures. The skull protects the brain; the vertebral column protects the spinal cord. The bony rib cage or thorax protects the heart, lungs, liver, spleen, stomach, and kidneys, whilst the pelvis looks after the bladder, colon, and female reproductive glands. Calcium is stored in the bones for use in the body when required.

FIGURE 1. The skeleton

Classification

Long bones consist of a shaft and two extremities or ends, e.g. the femur. The shaft is usually of compact bone, and the extremities are of cancellous bone surrounded with compact bone.

Short and irregular bones often consist mainly of cancellous tissue surrounded by a thin layer of compact bone and are short and irregular in shape and size, e.g. carpals, patella, vertebrae.

Flat bones are thin, flat, plate-like layers of compact bone sandwiched together with a filling of cancellous bone, e.g. scapulae, and bones of the skull and face.

There are certain features of the bones of the body which require particular mention, and for which there are special descriptive terms, devised and standardized by anatomists. Not only do these features present areas upon which the muscles are attached, or where joints articulate, but they may present bony points or places, over which massage may be contra-indicated, or where the beauty therapist must take special care.

TERMINOLOGY OF BONY FEATURES

Articular surface	smooth area for articulation with other bones
Facet	smooth area which may serve for articular surface
Condyle	smooth rounded prominence
Tuberosity	large prominence of bone rough or smooth
Tubercle	small or large depression in a bone
Foramen	a hole or opening in a bone
Spine	spiky bone (name given to the whole of the vertebral column)
Sulcus	groove or a furrow
Crest	a broad ridge or a sharp ridge
Process	a localized prominence
Hamulus	a hook-like process
Cornu	a horn-like process
Epicondyle	prominence above an articulating surface
Line	a long narrow ridge

ANATOMICAL POSITION

For purposes of all description the body is regarded as standing with the palms of the hand, as well as the chin and feet, facing forwards. This is called the *anatomical position*.

The midline of the body is taken as a line drawn down the centre of the vertebrae. It is from the anatomical position and the midline of the body that the following terminology of positions has been derived.

TERMINOLOGY OF POSITIONS

Anterior	in front of
Posterior	behind
Lateral	all that is away from the midline of the body
Medial	all that is nearest to midline
Lateral	(exterior medial) side of
Medial	(interior medial) inside of
Superior	above
Inferior	below
Proximal	near to the heart taking the heart as superior, e.g. upper arm is described as proximal
Distal	furthest away from the heart, e.g. lower arm or forearm is described as distal
Volar	anterior surface
Plantar	anterior, front surface (sole of foot is the plantar surface)
Dorsal	posterior, back surface (top of foot is the dorsum or dorsal surface)

The Extremities and Girdles of the Body

The upper and lower extremities of the body are attached to the trunk by bones and muscles. In the upper limb the bones which serve for attachment are the scapula and clavicle, and these, together with muscles, form the shoulder girdle (Figure 2). In front, the shoulder girdle articulates with the sternum by means of the clavicle, but behind, it only connects to the trunk by means of muscles from the scapula. The bones which connect the lower limb to the trunk are the hip bones (os innominata). At the front these two bones fuse together at the symphesis pubis. Behind, unlike the scapula, the gap between is filled in by the base of the sacrum with which the two hip bones articulate. This girdle of bones is called the pelvic girdle (Figure 3) and is a much stronger and more rigid construction than the lightweight shoulder girdle.

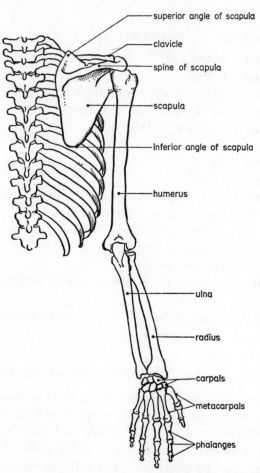

FIGURE 2. The right shoulder girdle

Both the upper and lower limbs are often referred to as the arms and legs. In anatomy the arm and leg sometimes refers only to certain parts of these extremities. They are divided as follows:

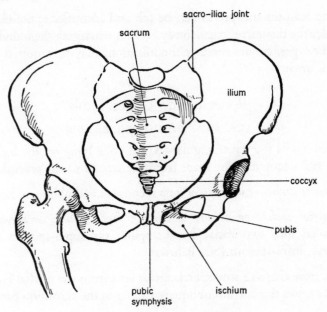

FIGURE 3. The female pelvic girdle

BONES OF THE UPPER LIMB (EXTREMITY)

Shoulder joint
Arm   (upper arm)
Elbow joint
Forearm   (lower arm)
Wrist
Hand   (and fingers)

BONES OF THE LOWER LIMB (EXTREMITY)

Hip joint
Thigh   (upper leg)
Knee joint
Leg   (lower leg)
Ankle joint
Foot   (and toes)

Major features and bony prominences of the bones which are of importance to the beauty therapist will be described. Some of these features and points can be felt and identified quite clearly under the tissues, subcutaneously. Whilst massaging the individual body types, certain massage modifications may be required over these areas.

Bones of the Upper Limb
SCAPULA (SHOULDER BLADE)

The scapula is a flat triangular-shaped bone lying on the back of the ribs occupying the space from the second to the seventh rib.

Anterior surface or subscapular fossa is concave and obliquely ridged.

Posterior surface or dorsum is convex from above downwards, divided into two fossae by the spine: the supra-spinous fossa above, infra-spinous fossa below.

The spine rises as a smooth triangular area from the medial border and crosses the dorsum obliquely ending in the acromion process.

Acromion process overhangs the glenoid cavity and articulates with the clavicle by a small facet on the inner border.

Three borders: Superior or Upper, Lateral or Axillary, and Medial or Vertebral.

Three angles: Superior, Inferior, and External, or Lateral. Lateral angle forms the Head and Neck of the scapula.

Head is the glenoid cavity for articulation with the head of the humerus, with a supra- and infra-glenoid tubercle.

Neck is the constriction immediately below the head.

Coracoid process lies on the upper border of the scapula above the head. When the arms are by the sides the coracoid process can be felt jutting forward immediately under the outer third of the clavicle. It is very painful when pressure is applied.

CLAVICLE (COLLAR BONE)

The clavicle is an irregular bone situated almost horizontally at the upper and anterior part of the thorax. It has a double curve being convex forward at the inner or medial end, and concave forward at the lateral or outer end.

It is divided into two parts for purposes of description for the beauty therapist:

Outer Third or flattened position.
Inner Third or prismatic portion.

The Two Ends are:

Sternal End with two facets.
Acromial End with one facet.

HUMERUS (UPPER ARM BONE)

The humerus is a long bone with a shaft and two extremities, an upper and lower extremity.

UPPER EXTREMITY

Head which is almost semispherical and directed upwards and inwards.

Anatomical neck which is a constriction in the bone immediately below the head.

Great tuberosity is large and lies uppermost and outermost.

Lesser tuberosity is small and lies on the inner side, separated from the great tuberosity by the bicipital groove, lying between the two tuberosities.

Surgical neck is the constriction of bone below the tuberosities and joins the shaft. It is the most common place for fractures of the humerus.

The shaft is cylindrical above but flattens out below, in front and behind.

LOWER EXTREMITY

The lower extremity is flattened posteriorly and convex anteriorly.

Two articulating surfaces which are the capitellum and trochlea.

Three fossae which are the coronoid fossa, olecranon fossa, and radial fossa.

Two condyles

Internal or Medial Condyle is the most prominent.

External or Lateral Condyle is fairly flat and round.

ULNA (INSIDE FOREARM BONE)

The ulna is a long bone lying on the inner side of the forearm. It has a shaft and two extremities.

UPPER EXTREMITY

The upper extremity is formed by two curved processes which are shaped to fit and articulate with the humerus. It also articulates with the radius.

Olecranon process curves forwards from the back of the ulna and hooks into the olecranon fossa of the humerus on extension.

Coronoid process projects upwards and forwards from the front of the ulna, hooking into the coronoid fossa of the humerus on flexion.

The two processes are continuous with the shaft.

THE SHAFT

The shaft is prismatic.

LOWER EXTREMITY

This consists of the head and styloid process.

The head is a rounded articular eminence on the lateral side of the shaft.

The styloid process lies medially and projects from the head; it is at a higher level than that of the radius.

RADIUS

The radius (outside forearm bone) is a long bone but shorter than the ulna; it lies on the outer side of the forearm playing a small part in the elbow joint, but a large part in the wrist. The two bones are connected by an inter-osseous membrane. This membrane deserves special mention because it has a poor blood supply. Therefore the beauty therapist must take care to finger knead thoroughly between these two bones when massaging the forearm in order to promote a good blood supply.

The radius has a shaft and two extremities.

UPPER EXTREMITY

The head is cylindrical.

The neck is the constricted part beneath the head.

Tuberosity (radial or bicipital) lies medially below the neck.

THE SHAFT

The shaft is prismatic and is slightly bowed outward.

LOWER EXTREMITY

The lower extremity is broad and triangular and articulates medially with the ulna.

Styloid process projects laterally and is lower than that of the ulna.

THE CARPUS (PALM BONES)

The carpus consists of eight small short bones arranged in two rows. There are four in each of the proximal and distal rows. The pisiform bone is the most easily palpated bone, lying just above the hypothenar eminence of the palm; and the scaphoid can be felt above the thenar eminence on the lateral side of the palm. The other carpus can be more easily felt through the skin on the posterior surface of the hand, particularly as the carpus is convex here.

Each name describes the shape or the position of the bone. They all fit together like pieces of crazy paving.

Proximal row from lateral to medial side:

Scaphoid	boat-shaped
Lunate	crescent-shaped
Triquetral	three-sided
Pisiform	pea-shaped

Distal row lateral to medial side:

Trapezium	four-sided, with two parallel sides (the larger bone)
Trapezoid	four-sided, with no parallel sides (the smaller bone)
Capitate	has a head and is the largest carpal
Hamate	hook-like

METACARPUS (HAND BONES)

There are five metacarpal bones numbered from the lateral to the medial side. They are small long bones, possessing a shaft and two extremities, the head and base. The head is rounded and the base is flattened out, articulating with the carpus. The head can be felt as the knuckles on the dorsum of the hand. The first metacarpal, that of the thumb, does not lie alongside the other four. Because of its position it is able to move medially in front of the palm when it is flexed, and is a most important factor in increasing gripping power. This is called opposition.

First metacarpal is shorter and stronger than the others.

Second and third metacarpal are usually the longest.

Fourth metacarpal is more slender than the others.

Fifth metacarpal is the smallest.

PHALANGES (FINGER BONES, OR DIGITS)

There are *fourteen* in number, two for the thumb and three for each finger. Each has a head, shaft, and base or proximal end. In each, the shaft tapers to its distal end. The distal phalanges taper to a fine, slim, non-articulating head.

Bones of the Lower Limb (Leg)

See Figure 4.

FIGURE 4. The bones of the right leg

OS INNOMINATUM (HIP BONE)

This bone consists of three united bones, which are the ilium, ischium, and pubis. The junction of these bones forms the cup-like depression in the hip bone called the acetabulum, which articulates with the head of the femur and so forms the hip joint.

ILIUM

The main bony point to be considered as far as the beauty therapist is concerned is the upper border of the ilium, referred to frequently as the *iliac crest*.

Iliac crest. The most palpable portion of the crest is situated anteriorly just below the waist and is called the anterior iliac spine. There is a superior and inferior iliac spine. This lip-like crest sweeps upwards and backwards to end in the posterior superior spine articulating with the sacrum. The crest provides an attachment place for several muscles, the bony surface being rough and stressed.

ISCHIUM

This projects backwards and consists of the body, ramus, and tuberosity. It is the ischial tuberosity that can be felt through thick and thin after having been seated too long on a hard seat. The beauty therapist should ensure the comfort of the client with an extra pillow if she is to be treated in a sitting position for any length of time.

PUBIS

The pubis consists of a body, superior, and inferior ramus, none of which can be palpated, except for the superior ramus which projects forwards to the midline of the body and articulates with the pubic bone of the opposite side.

Obturator foramen is a hole in the os innominatum between the ischium and pubis. It is oval in the male, and triangular in the female.

FEMUR (THIGH BONE)

This is the longest and largest bone in the body. It is also reputed to be the strongest. It slopes obliquely downwards and inwards, being farther apart at the hip joints and nearer together at the knee joints. Like the other long bones it has a shaft and two extremities.

UPPER EXTREMITY

The upper extremity presents the head which is almost spherical, being directed upwards, inwards, and slightly forwards, and articulates with the acetabulum.

Neck connects the head to the shaft at an angle of 125°.

Great trochanter. This is a large four-sided prominence, situated at the upper and outer part of the function of the neck with the shaft. It is the area over which fatty deposits seem to be the most stubborn to reduce. It is to this great trochanter that many women women can attribute their 'pear-shaped' figure, widening from the waist downwards and outwards, depending upon size and shape of this particular part of the bone.

The lesser trochanter lies medially at the posterior part of the neck and cannot be felt.

Tubercle lies between the great trochanter and lesser trochanter, and the gluteal ridge lies posteriorly below the great trochanter.

SHAFT

This is almost cylindrical, being smooth anteriorly but strengthened behind by a prominent ridge along and into which several muscles are attached.

LOWER EXTREMITY

The lower extremity consists of two condyles. Behind, between the two, lies the inter-condylar notch. In front is the patella surface. The inferior and posterior surfaces of the condyles articulate with the tibia to form the knee joint.

Internal Condyle is longer than the external when the bone is vertical.

External Condyle is wider than the internal condyle.

TIBIA (LARGE INSIDE LEG BONE)

The tibia is situated at the front and inner side of the leg. It is the second largest bone in the body. It consists of a shaft and two extremities.

UPPER EXTREMITY

The upper extremity is expanded into two condyles. The anterior sides of the condyles make a continuous surface. The posterior surface is separated by the popliteal notch, and its superior articulating surface is centred by a roughened raised area called the spine. In front of and below the tibial condyles, projecting forwards between them, lies the *tibial tubercle*. This raised 'bump' can easily be felt, especially when the knee is flexed.

Medial Condyle is larger than the lateral.

Lateral Condyle overhangs the shaft but presents a small surface for articulation with the fibula.

SHAFT

The shaft is triangular and has three borders and three surfaces.

The anterior border and medial surface is subcutaneous, and is usually referred to as the 'shin'. Great care is essential when finger kneading in this area, between the tibia and fibula.

LOWER EXTREMITY

The lower end of the tibia is expanded into several portions, its medial portion projecting lower than the rest of the bone, and is called the medial malleolus.

Medial malleolus is short and strong, and can be felt very easily through the skin. It is sometimes referred to as the ankle bone.

FIBULA (THIN OUTSIDE LEG BONE)

This is a slender long bone, and lies on the lateral side of the leg. It has a *head*, its upper end, which can be palpated quite easily just below the lateral side of the knee and which articulates with the tibia. It has a *shaft*, and a lower end, the *lateral malleolus*, or the outside ankle bone, which projects lower than the medial malleolus of the tibia.

PATELLA (KNEE BONE)

The patella is the largest sesamoid bone (or a bone that lies in a tendon). It lies in front of the knee joint in the quadriceps tendon. It is flat and triangular and can be easily palpated and passively moved. Deep finger kneadings and frictions around the patella are advocated in a detailed body massage.

TARSUS (FOREFOOT BONES)

There are seven tarsi comparable to the carpi of the hand, but much larger and stronger because of their function in the body (Figure 5). They are arranged in two rows:

Proximal row consists of the talus, calcaneum (heel bone), and navicular.

Distal row consists of three cuneiform bones and the cuboid.

FIGURE 5.   The bones of the foot

Talus lies slightly above and to the front of the calcaneum. It supports the tibia and articulates on either side with the malleoli, and in front with the scaphoid. It can be felt quite easily projecting forwards at the front of the ankle.

Calcaneum (heel bone) is the largest of the tarsal bones. It transmits the weight of the body to the ground, articulating with the talus and the cuboid bones. It can be felt as the bony heel.

Navicular bone is situated in the medial part of the tarsus and articulates with the three cuneiform bones. It can be felt through the skin below the medial malleolus.

Cuboid is the most lateral bone in the distal row of the tarsus. It lies between the calcaneum, the outer two metatarsal bones.

Cuneiform bones articulate in front with the three inner metatarsals, behind with the navicular bone, and with each other lying side by side.

Medial Cuneiform is the largest.

Middle Cuneiform is the smallest and wedge-shaped.

Lateral Cuneiform articulates with six bones.

THE METATARSUS (MID-FOOT BONES)

These bones, like the metacarpi, are mini-long bones. There are five in number and they are situated in the anterior part of the foot in front of the tarsus. They are numbered from the medial to the lateral side. They comprise a head (distal end), base (proximal end), and a shaft.

The heads articulate with the proximal row of the phalanges, and the bases articulate with the distal row of the tarsus.

First metatarsal is shortest and thickest with a strong body.

Second metatarsal is longest and has a wedge-shaped base.

Third metatarsal has a triangular-shaped base.

Fourth metatarsal is shorter than the third.

Fifth metatarsal has a tubercle which can be palpated on the lateral side of its base.

PHALANGES (TOE BONES)

There are fourteen in number and they correspond in general arrangement with those of the hand. There is a proximal, middle, and distal row. The middle row are remarkably short and small, but broader than the proximal row. The distal phalanges are much smaller than those in the fingers, and each has a rough tuberosity on its plantar aspect.

The Vertebral Column (Back Bones)

There are thirty-three vertebrae in the vertebral column. The column is made up of seven cervical, twelve thoracic, five lumbar, five sacral, and four coccygeal vertebrae. Between each vertebra there is a cartilaginous disk which sometimes acts as a shock absorber for harsh movements, except in the sacral and coccygeal bones which are fused together. Each group of vertebrae, whilst having individual characteristics, is generally constructed on the same lines, and becomes progressively stronger and heavier from the cervical region downwards. The vertebral column is often referred to as the spine. This name is derived from the spinous processes which are common to nearly all the bones. They can be felt quite easily down the centre of the back, and it is these particular bony prominences over which great care should be taken when massaging the back, in particular when applying frictions and finger kneadings either side of the spine, for it can be excruciatingly painful. The vertebral column or spine provides the body with its central axis round which, and from which, all movements take place. It also serves to protect the spinal cord and it supports the weight of the trunk, transmitting it through to the lower limbs.

A typical vertebra (Figure 6) is made up of a fat anterior chunk of bone called the body, behind which lies a canal which contains the spinal cord. The spinal cord is the extension of the brain and is part of the central nervous system of the body, extending from the first cervical vertebra to the first lumber vertebra where it begins to taper off down into the coccyx. It is surrounded by the formation of two thin backward projecting bars of bone, extending from the body called the pedicles. The laminae extend from the pedicles and unite to form the spinous process which projects sideways. There are articulating facets on the vertebrae above and below for articulation with each other. The first and second vertebrae are called the atlas and axis. Nodding and shaking of the head is made possible by the construction of these two bones and their joints.

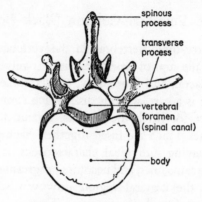

FIGURE 6. A typical vertebra

The thoracic vertebrae only articulate with the ribs. In the lumbar region the spines of the vertebrae are almost horizontally directed, and they are much larger than all the other vertebrae.

The sacrum is a triangular wedge-shaped bone. Its apex is at the inferior end of the bone, and articulates with the two hip bones, into and around which joint finger kneadings and frictions prove to be most beneficial. The *coccyx* is the rudimentary tail of Man and curves downwards and forwards from the apex of the sacrum, deep between the gluteal fold of muscle.

CURVES OF THE VERTEBRAL COLUMN

There are four curves of the spine. Those in the thoracic and pelvic region are known as the primary curves, and are formed before birth, remaining constant after. Those of the cervical and lumbar region are only formed later after birth as the child sits and then walks. These are called the secondary curves. The cervical curve is convex forwards; the thoracic curve is concave forwards; the lumbar curve is convex forwards and the pelvic curve formed by the sacrum and coccyx, is concave forwards. Any deviation from these normal curves, generally due to poor posture, overweight, or lack of exercise, can cause deformities of the spine. Compensatory effects, causing added stress and strain throughout the body, will occur sooner or later.

THE STERNUM (BREAST BONE)

The sternum is a long flat bone lying in the middle and upper part of the anterior wall of the thorax. It consists of the broad *manubrium* above which articulates with the sternal end of the clavicle. It has a *body* which extends from the manubrium downwards and is fairly broad and convex in front, tapering to the *xiphoid process* below. The whole of the sternum articulates on either side with the first seven pairs of ribs. It is an extremely uncomfortable bone to have massaged and only the lightest of work is performed over and around it.

THE RIBS

Gray's 'Anatomy' describes a rib as being an 'elastic arch' of bone. There are twelve ribs at each side of the vertebral column, with which they articulate. In front, the first seven pairs only are connected by cartilage to and articulate with the sternum. These are called true ribs, while the remaining five are called false ribs. The eighth, ninth, and tenth ribs are each joined, again by cartilage, to the rib above, whilst the eleventh and twelfth are free in front and known as floating ribs. Together with the thoracic vertebrae and the sternum the twelve pairs of ribs form the thorax, or rib cage.

The thorax is a conical-shaped cage of bone and cartilage, protecting mainly the heart and the lungs. Because of the varying shapes of the ribs, it is narrow above, flat from front to back, gradually increasing in size, from the first to the seventh rib, from side to side, decreasing and tapering from the seventh rib, to become longer behind at the twelfth rib than in front.

A typical rib (Figure 7) has a head, neck, tubercle, angle, and shaft. The head and tubercle articulate with the body and the transverse process of the corresponding vertebra. The head also articulates with the vertebra above. From the angle of the rib, it is bent forward and twisted. The intercostal muscles are attached between the ribs.

FIGURE 7.   A typical rib

On a thin person, massage over the anterior parts of the rib cage would be restricted to kneading or ironing. This applies to the back of the rib cage. Sometimes finger kneadings are applied to the intercostal muscles in conditions such as fibrositis, but this very often proves to be a ticklish and impossible job. It is around the margins of the lower ribs (midriff) that adipose tissue seems to settle both in men and women, and it is more often than not that this spare tyre of flesh requires vigorous treatment in the form of wringing, picking up, and hacking.

THE SKULL

The skull (Figure 8) consists of several flat bones which are divided into the bones of the head (cranium) and the face. With the exception of the mandible, the joints of the skull are immovable. The upper part of the cranium forms a protective box around the brain, and it is often called the vortex of the skull, the lower part being called the base.

The forehead is composed of the *frontal bone* which extends backwards to meet the left and right parietal bones, which form the main part of the top of the head. These two bones, sutured together, extend backwards and unite with the *occipital bone* at the base of the skull. In front of the occiput and on either side can be found the *temporal bones*, which give rise to the *mastoid process* immediately palpated behind the earlobe.

parietal bone

frontal bone

orbit

temporal bone

nasal bones

zygomatic bone

mastoid process

maxilla

angle of jaw

mandible

FIGURE 8.   The skull

The temple is formed partly by the *temporal bones*, the other part being formed by the *sphenoid bones* sandwiched between the frontal above, and the *zygomatic bones* in front.

The cheek prominence is mainly formed by the zygomatic bones, which join up with the *maxillae*, forming the upper jaw and sides of the nose.

The nose mainly consists of the *nasal bones* which extend backwards into the orbits of the eyes, and these bones are called *ethmoid* and *lacrimal* bones.

The orbits of the eyes are two hollows formed by the shapes of the surrounding bones.

Foramen magnum is the name given to a large hole formed in the base of the skull, in the occipital bone. It is through this hole that the brain extends as the spinal cord, into the neural canal of the vertebrae.

THE MANDIBLE (LOWER JAW BONE)

The mandible is the large bone of the face. It consists of a body and a ramus which are easily identified on the living body.

The chin is formed by the fusion of the body of the left and right mandibles in midline. The triangular part of the chin is formed by the mental protuberance of either side. The lower border of the body extends backwards and forms the jawline of the face.

The angle of the jaw is formed by the fusion of the body with the ramus which extends upwards into a two-pronged fork-like projection. The anterior prong of the fork is called the coronoid process. The posterior prong extends into the head of the mandible which articulates with the temporal bone, forming the temporo-mandibular joint. Between the prong of bone is the mandibular notch. When the mouth is opened, the mandible being depressed, the coronoid process can easily be palpated. It is round this area that special care should be taken when massaging.

N.B. As the body grows older the mandible shrinks in size. This could be one reason for the tissues, skin muscle, and fat round this area becoming noticeably loose, and for the gradual disappearance of the firm contour of the jawline.

The hyoid bone lies immediately underneath the interior of the temporal bones. It is the bone of the throat and is wing-shaped.

7. Joints

The study of joints is called arthrology. When two or more skeletal structures meet they form a joint or an articulation. In flat bones, such as those of the skull, it is the edges which form the joints; in irregularly shaped bones such as the tarsals it can be anywhere on their surfaces which articulate; and in long bones it is usually their extremities which form the joints, such as in the femur. Bones are united in three different ways. Firstly, where movement is undesirable, the bones are united by fibrous tissue. Secondly, cartilage unites bones where a small degree of movement is necessary. Thirdly, where a large amount of movement is called for, the bones are united by a tough membrane called the capsule; this in turn is lined by the synovial membrane.

Classification

FIBROUS JOINTS

Fibrous joints are subdivided into two types:

Sutures, such as the immovable joints found in the skull, are joints where the bones are united by strips of fibrous tissue which are continuous with the periosteum.

Syndesmosis, such as the joints between the bones in the leg and forearm, where they are united by interosseus ligaments and membranes and where movement is very limited.

CARTILAGINOUS JOINTS

Cartilaginous joints are subdivided into two types:

Preliminary, such as can be found in growing bones. The bones are connected by a thin plate of cartilage which eventually becomes bone when the growth of the bone is complete. This kind of joint is only temporary and is quite fixed.

Secondary, such as the joints between the pubic bones called the symphesis pubis and between the bodies of the vertebrae. The movement is very limited in these joints and they are found in midline of the body.

SYNOVIAL JOINTS

Synovial joints are subdivided into six types. They are freely movable joints, and nearly all the joints of the body fall into this class. Certain structural characteristics are common throughout but their classification is according to mobility.

Hinge joint, such as the elbow joint, where the movement takes place round one axis (transverse axis) which is limited to flexion and extension.

Pivot joint, such as the joint between the head of the radius and the ulna, or between the first and second cervical vertebrae (atlas and axis). Again the movement takes place round one axis (longitudinal axis) and is a rotatory movement.

Condyloid joint, such as the metacarpo-phalangeal joints of the fingers, the movements taking place round two axes, a horizontal and sagittal axis and consisting of flexion, extension, abduction, and adduction but no rotation.

Saddle joint, such as the carpo-metacarpo joint of the thumb, where the shape of the articulating surfaces can be likened to two inverted saddles being placed over each other at right angles. Here again the movements are bi-axial producing flexion, extension, abduction, adduction, and a combination of those four movements which is called circumduction.

Ball and socket joint, such as the hip joint where the almost spherical head of one bone fits into the cup-shaped depression of another. The extensive movements take place round an indefinite number of axes, consisting of flexion, extension, abduction, adduction, rotation, and circumduction.

Gliding joint, such as the joints between the tarsal bones in the foot and the carpal bones at the wrist. It is formed by the opposition of plane surfaces, and the gliding movement produced has no definite axis.

STRUCTURES OF A TYPICAL SYNOVIAL JOINT

BONES

Bones, which are covered on their articulating surfaces with hyaline cartilage. The elastic hyaline cartilage provides strength, allowing frictionless and painless movement. It has no blood or nerve supply and obtains its nourishment from the fluid of the synovial membrane.

JOINT CAPSULE

The joint capsule is the sheath of fibrous tissue uniting the two bones creating a joint cavity. The capsule is very often reinforced by strong bands of fibrous tissue which usually blend with the periosteum.

SYNOVIAL MEMBRANE

The synovial membrane (Figure 9) lines the capsule and sometimes passes into the joint cavity over the hyaline cartilage. It secretes a fluid which, as well as providing food for the bone ends, lubricates the hyaline cartilage assisting its smooth movement. If the synovial membrane becomes inflamed (synovitis) there is an increase of synovial fluid into and around the joint. It becomes painful and swollen.

LIGAMENTS

Ligaments are of strong interlaced bundles of fibrous tissue. Although they are pliant they are inextensible so that they do not stretch. The direction of these fibres depends upon the stress which is put on the joint, and they are known as the accessory ligaments. Further ligaments can be found inside the capsule

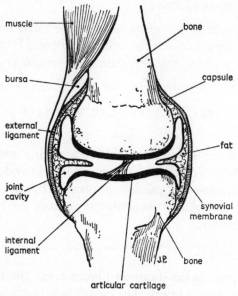

FIGURE 9.   A synovial joint

uniting the articular surfaces, and ligaments which deepen the articulating depression can be found in the shoulder and hip joint.

ARTICULAR DISKS

Articular disks may be found between the articulating surfaces.

MUSCLES

Muscles representing the power of the joint pass over one or two joints producing movement, often stabilizing the joint against gravity. Sometimes, between the joint capsule and the muscle, small fibrous sacs filled with synovial fluid can be found. These are called bursae and act as cushions to prevent friction.

BLOOD VESSELS

Blood vessels bring nourishment to the joint structures and so enable them to function normally.

NERVES

Nerves from the muscles which act upon the joints convey the sensory impressions to the brain from the joints, so that the brain is aware of what action the joint is taking.

FATTY PADS

Fatty pads can be found inside the joint filling in the crevices.

MOVEMENTS WHICH TAKE PLACE IN JOINTS

The movements which take place in joints can be divided into four categories. They are gliding, angular, rotatory, and circumductory. Very often it can be found that most joints are capable of producing a variety of movements. When the articulating surfaces of the bones are reduced in size the range of movement is likely to be restricted. When they are greater in size then the range of movement will be increased, particularly on the more movable bone. The fundamental anatomical starting position, unless otherwise stated, will be used when describing the following movements:

ANGULAR MOVEMENTS

Angular movement produces an increase or decrease of the angle between the two bones. It consists of two movements which take place around axes set at right angles to each other. The movements are called flexion coupled with extension, and abduction with adduction.

FLEXION

Flexion is generally understood to mean the decreasing of the angle between two bones. This could be called bending. Extension is the opposite movement and could be called straightening. Bending the trunk forwards is an example of flexion in the vertebrae. Standing up straight produces extension in these joints. Flexion at the ankle joint brings the dorsum of the foot up towards the leg; this is called dorsiflexion. When the foot is stretched downwards from the ankle joint in extension it is termed plantarflexion. Flexion of the shoulder joint results in the arm being carried forwards, upwards, and medially. Flexion at the knee joint results in the leg being drawn backwards, towards, and approaching the back of the thigh.

LATERAL FLEXION

Lateral flexion or side flexion is the term given to the movement of the vertebral column when any part of it bends sideways, either at the waist (lumbar region) or neck (cervical region) or in the more restricted middle back (thoracic region).

EVERSION

Eversion is the term used when the joints of the foot turn the sole of the foot to face sideways (laterally).

INVERSION

Inversion is the term used to describe the movement of the foot when the sole of the foot is turned to face inwards (medially).

ABDUCTION

Abduction is a movement which carries the limbs away from the middle of the body, which is taken as a line drawn down the centre of the vertebrae. The fingers move away from the midline of the middle finger.

ADDUCTION

Adduction is the movement towards midline of the body, or the fingers to the middle finger.

ELEVATION

Elevation is the term used to describe the movements taking place in the shoulder girdle. When the arm is abducted to shoulder level the movement which takes the arm from this point up towards the side of the head and ear is termed elevation through abduction. When the arm is flexed to shoulder level, the movement which takes the arm upwards to the side of the head and ear is termed elevation through flexion.

DEPRESSION

Depression is the term used to describe the movement of the temporo-mandibular joint when the mouth is opened.

ROTATION

Rotation is a movement in which the bone moves round its long axis, as in the femur when the lower limb is turned either medially inwards or laterally outwards (medial and lateral rotation). Rotation can also take place when one bone pivots round another as in the atlanto-axial joint, which results in turning the head and chin to the left or right. Rotation of the radius round the ulna turns the palm of the hand to face backwards. This is called pronation. When the palm of the hand is turned to face forwards as in the anatomical position this is called supination. These two movements are best illustrated when the elbow is semiflexed. The palm of the hand when facing upwards is supinated and when turned downwards is pronated. Thus prone lying is lying face and anterior surface downwards. Lying supine means lying face upwards, and lying on the posterior surface of the body (on the back).

CIRCUMDUCTION

Circumduction presents a combination of the four angular movements. The bone describes the shape of a cone with the apex of the cone at the joint. The hip and shoulder joints are good examples for this kind of movement, in which large circles of movement can be performed.

FACTORS WHICH STABILIZE AND RESTRICT JOINT MOVEMENT

The stability and safety of the joints rely on several factors which limit movement. The tension of ligaments and muscles is very important in preventing excess movement in any one direction, which might strain the joint. Once a ligament has been torn or stretched it is difficult to fully repair. The stability of the joint can therefore be affected and so it is primarily the tone of the muscles which helps to prevent overstretching of the ligaments, and can restrict joint movement. It is only the perfect balance of tone between the opposing postural muscle groups that keeps the body in the erect and upright position. No other factors play a part in stabilizing the joints in this normal position. The shape and size of the articular facets can restrict movement. On movement, contact with other bones and soft structures is another prohibiting factor, e.g. on flexion of the hip joint, the thigh comes into contact with the abdominal wall. The movement is therefore halted and active overstretching prevented. Tension of the capsule of the joint produces a reflex contraction in the opposing muscle group to that which is moving the joint. This in turn again prevents overstretching and tearing of the joint structures. Poor posture and lack of tone in postural muscles can lead to stress and strain on one or more joints of the body. This can be a contributory factor in the cause of arthritic conditions, wear and tear of cartilages and disks, and many more diseases of the joints and their structures.

However, ligaments, as well as inadvertently being overstretched, can be deliberately relaxed in order to produce a wider range of joint movement for a specific purpose, such as in sports, ballet, yoga, and even in exercising the hands and fingers to make them more supple for massage.

Joints of the Upper Limb

STERNO-CLAVICULAR JOINT

Between the sternum and the clavicle.

Type: synovial.

ACROMIO-CLAVICULAR JOINT

Between the acromion process of the scapula and the clavicle.

Type: synovial.

MOVEMENTS

These two joints make up the joints of the shoulder girdle. The movement permitted in them is a slight gliding movement when the scapula moves.

Elevation and depression of the scapula—shrugging up and down of the shoulder girdle muscles.

Rotation forwards and retraction backwards of the scapula round the chest wall—as in punching and pushing forwards, and bracing the shoulder girdle backwards.

Rotation upwards and downwards of the scapula—as when the arm is raised above the head and brought down again. This movement involves movement in the shoulder joint.

SHOULDER JOINT

Between the head of the humerus and the glenoid cavity of the scapula.

Type: ball and socket.

MOVEMENTS

Flexion: the arm is brought upwards forwards and slightly medially across the chest.

Extension: the arm is drawn downwards and backwards behind the trunk.

Abduction: the arm is raised sideways to shoulder level away from midline of the body.

Adduction: the arm is drawn down towards midline of the body and side of the trunk.

Medial or inward rotation: the hand is turned inwards and round towards the body as far as possible so that the palms face backwards.

Outward or lateral rotation: the hand is turned outwards as far as possible so that the palm faces laterally and sideways.

Elevation is a movement of the shoulder girdle which is the movement of the arm above the head from shoulder level, either taking it up through flexion or abduction.

Circumduction is the circling round of the arm which can take place when all the above movements are combined together. The hand can describe a huge cone, the apex of the cone being at the shoulder joint.

ELBOW JOINT

Between humerus and ulna, and the humerus and radius.

Type: hinge joint.

MOVEMENTS

Flexion: the forearm is bent up towards the upper arm.

Extension: the forearm is stretched away from the upper arm straightening out. Because of the shape of the lower end of the humerus when the forearm is extended it does not lie in a straight line with the upper arm. It is displaced laterally away from the body at an angle to the upper arm. This angle is called the 'carrying' angle. It is said to have acquired this name because of the way in which heavy loads are carried away from the side, in order to avoid bumping the body.

RADIO-ULNAR JOINTS

Superior and inferior joints between the upper and lower ends of the radius and ulna (and a connection between the two bones by an interosseus membrane).

Type: synovial and pivot joints.

MOVEMENTS

See Figure 10.

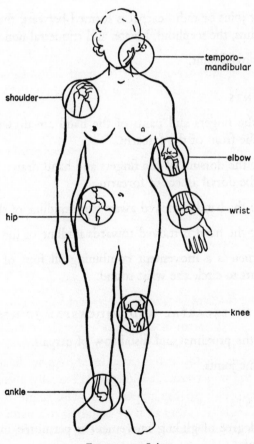

temporo-
mandibular

shoulder

elbow

hip

wrist

knee

ankle

FIGURE 10. Joints

Pronation is a movement of the radius which turns the palm from its anatomical position (palm when facing upwards), when the elbow is semi-flexed, downwards.

Supination is a corkscrew-like movement which turns the palm, when the elbow is semi-flexed, upwards. Pronation and supination are movements that can be confused with medial and lateral (outward) rotation of the shoulder joint if performed when the arm is by the side.

WRIST JOINT

The wrist joint or radio-carpal is formed between the distal end of the radius, the scaphoid, lunate, and triquetral bones.

Type: synovial joint.

MOVEMENTS

Flexion: the fingers and palm of the hand are drawn forwards towards the front of the forearm.

Extension: the dorsum of the fingers and hand drawn backwards towards the dorsal aspect of forearm.

Abduction: the hand is moved away from midline of the body.

Adduction: the hand is moved towards midline of the body.

Circumduction is a movement combining all four of the above movements to circle the wrist round.

INTERCARPAL AND MIDCARPAL JOINTS

Between the proximal and distal row of carpals.

Type: plane joints.

MOVEMENTS

A small degree of gliding movement is permitted in the intercarpal joints.

Flexion, extension, abduction, and adduction of the mid-carpal joints in conjunction with the wrist and fingers.

CARPO-METACARPAL JOINT OF THE THUMB

Between trapezium and first metacarpal bones.

Type: saddle joint.

MOVEMENTS

Flexion of the thumb results in a sideways movement across the palm of the hand and is combined with opposition, in which the thumb can stretch over to the base of the other four fingers. There is also a slight degree of rotation.

Extension takes the thumb out sideways away from the palm.

Abduction takes the thumb forwards and at right angles to the palm of the hand.

Adduction brings the thumb back to the side of the hand.

Circumduction is a combination of all the above movements of the thumb circling it round.

CARPO-METACARPAL JOINTS OF FINGERS

These are between the carpals and metacarpal bones of the second, third, fourth, and fifth metacarpals.

Type: plane joint.

Movements: gliding.

INTERMETACARPAL JOINTS

These are between the metacarpal bones and joined together by interosseus ligaments.

Type: synovial.

Movement: gliding.

METACARPO-PHALANGEAL JOINTS

These joints (knuckles) are between the metacarpal bones and the bases of the proximal phalanges.

Type: condyloid.

MOVEMENTS

Flexion bends the fingers into the palm from the knuckle.

Extension straightens them back in line with the palm.

Abduction takes the index, ring, and little finger away from the midline of the middle finger.

Adduction brings them back towards the midline.

Circumduction: circular movement combining the four angular movements.

INTERPHALANGEAL JOINTS

Between the phalanges.

Type: hinge joints.

MOVEMENTS

Flexion is a movement of bending the fingers towards the palm of the hand.

Extension is the opposite movement of straightening and stretching the fingers backwards away from the palm of the hand.

Joints of the Lower Limb

PUBIC-SYMPHESIS JOINT

Between the two pubic bones.

Type: secondary cartilaginous.

Movements: limited movement, except in pregnancy when relaxation of the ligaments allows greater freedom of movement.

HIP JOINT

Between the head of the femur and the acetabulum of the os innominata bone.

Type: ball and socket.

MOVEMENTS

Flexion draws the thigh up on to the abdominal wall.

Extension takes the thigh from flexion downwards away from the abdominal wall and backwards towards the posterior aspect of the trunk.

Abduction carries the leg away from midline of the body sideways.

Adduction carries the leg in towards midline of the body.

Medial rotation (*inward*) turns the whole lower limb inwards from the hip.

Lateral rotation (*outward*) is the movement which turns the whole lower limb out.

Circumduction—is a combination of all the above movements in a circular motion.

KNEE JOINT

Between the condyles of the femur and tibia, and an articulation between the patella and femur.

Type: hinge joint.

MOVEMENTS

Flexion bends the leg backwards to the back of the thigh.

Extension draws the leg straight forwards in a line with the thigh.

Medial rotation at the knee joint occurs mainly when the knee is semi-flexed and involves a small inward turning of the leg on the thigh.

Lateral rotation occurs mainly when the knee is semi-flexed and turns the leg slightly outwards on the thigh.

Gliding occurs slightly with the patella and femur.

ANKLE JOINT

Between the bones of the lower end of the tibia, fibula, and talus.

Type: hinge joint.

MOVEMENTS

Dorsiflexion: the foot and toes are pulled upwards towards the front surface of the leg.

Plantarflexion: the foot and toes are pointed downwards.

Gliding movements are possible.

INTERTARSAL JOINTS

Formed between the bones of:

(a) calcaneum and talus　　(b) cuneiform bones and navicular
(c) calcaneum and cuboid　(d) cuneiform bones
(e) cuboid and navicular　　(f) inter-cuneiform
(g) cuneiform and cuboid

Types: (a) plane; (b) ball and socket; (c) saddle; (d) plane; (e) plane; (f) plane; (g) plane.

MOVEMENTS

Gliding of the bones on each other intensifies the flexibility of the foot.

Rotation occurs on inversion and eversion.

Inversion: the sole of the foot (plantar surface) is turned to face inwards.

Eversion: the plantar surface of the foot is turned to face outwards.

TARSAL AND METATARSAL JOINT

Between the cuneiform, cuboid, and metatarsal bones.

Type: plane.

Movement: gliding.

INTERMETATARSAL JOINTS

Between the metatarsal bones.

Type: syndesmosis.

Movement: slight gliding movement.

METATARSO-PHALANGEAL JOINTS

Between the metatarsal and proximal phalanges.

Type: condyloid.

MOVEMENTS

Flexion: toes are bent downwards and forwards.

Extension: toes are stretched upwards and backwards.

Abduction: the big toe, third, fourth, and fifth toes move away from the second toe.

Adduction: the big toe, third, fourth, and fifth toes move toward the second toe.

INTERPHALANGEAL JOINTS

Between the phalanges.
Type: hinge joint.

MOVEMENTS

Flexion: curling the toes over and down.

Extension: uncurling and straightening the toes.

JOINTS OF THE VERTEBRAL COLUMN

As a whole are between the bodies and arches of the vertebrae.

Type: cartilaginous and plane.

MOVEMENTS

Flexion: forward bending of the head and trunk.

Extension is a backward stretching and arching.

Lateral flexion (side-flexion): sideways bending of the head and trunk.

Rotation is a movement which turns the trunk from side to side.

JOINTS OF THE RIBS

These are between the bones of the ribs and corresponding vertebrae posteriorly, and the ribs and sternum anteriorly.

Type: synovial.

MOVEMENTS

The movement of the ribs is brought about by the mechanism of respiration, when the lungs take in air and expand on inspiration. The thorax or rib cage increases all round in size, rather like opening a venetian blind. The sternum is pushed forwards at the same time. On expiration the rib cage collapses, the size of the thorax being decreased again as the air is driven out of the lungs.

SACRO-ILIAC JOINT

Between the sacrum and ilium bone at the base of the spine.

Type: plane joint.

MOVEMENTS

Very little movement takes place in the sacro-iliac joint normally but a little interplay between the bones is permitted. The joint surfaces lock into each other on movements such as jumping and act as a shock absorber together with the cartilaginous disks between the bodies of the other vertebrae. During pregnancy and childbirth the range of movement at this joint increases to allow more room and greater mobility in the pelvis. However, as the body ages, this joint stiffens and fuses together, mobility being lost. It is a common area for chronic backache. The joint itself is one which can be strained, together with the joints in the lumbar region, especially if poor posture and the wrong standing position is adopted, for both young and old alike.

JOINTS OF THE SKULL

These are between the bones of the cranium and are called sutures; there is no movement between them.

Coronal suture: between the frontal and parietal bones runs across from side to side of the skull.

Sagittal suture: between the two parietal bones, runs from the front to the back of the skull.

Lamboid suture: between the parietal and occipital bones, runs downwards and forwards at the back of the skull.

TEMPORO-MANDIBULAR JOINT

This joint (the jaw) is between the temporal and mandible bones.

Type: hinge joint.

MOVEMENTS

Depression: opening the mouth (mandible or jaw).

Elevation: closing the mouth (mandible or jaw).

Protrusion: jutting forward of the mandible.

Retraction: pulling backward of the mandible.

Lateral movement: sideways movement of the mandible as in chewing.

In many joints of the body, accessory (additional) movements to those described above can be found. One kind of accessory movement can be produced when an active movement is resisted, enabling another one to be produced. The movement permitted in the play between the articulating surfaces, which are themselves accessory movements during added stress and strain of a joint, is made use of in passive movements. These movements are performed on the relaxed muscles and joints by the beauty therapist. All active movements which are performed on the body are brought about by the action of specific muscles which pass over the joints.

8. *Muscles*

Myology is the name given to the study of muscles. Muscles are considered to be the meat and flesh of the body, and it is mainly the muscles of the body which are manipulated in massage. Not only is it important for the beauty therapist to know how the muscles lie in the body so that individual muscle or muscle groups can be treated and massaged correctly, but it is essential to know the name, origin, insertion, and action of the muscles if corrective and helpful schemes of exercises are to be planned, in conjunction with massage and a good diet. Every muscle in the body serves a purpose and has a function, but only the superficial individual muscles and muscle groups will be described. These can easily be identified on the living body.

Kinds of Muscular Tissue

There are three kinds of muscular tissue:

1. *Involuntary* which deals with actions over which we have no control and are not conscious of doing such as the alimentary tract.
2. *Cardiac*, the specialized muscle tissue of the heart.
3. *Voluntary* muscle tissue which deals with actions over which we have control and are conscious of doing. The beauty therapist is mainly concerned with the voluntary muscles of the body.

All the individual muscles of the body are made up of muscle fibres. The muscle fibres in turn are bound together in clusters by connective tissue, and the clusters are then connected into a large group to form an individual muscle. Sometimes individual muscles are bound together by fascia to form a muscle group. Each muscle has an origin and an insertion.

Characteristics of Muscle Fibres

ORIGIN

The origin of a muscle is normally its most fixed point of attachment, and is its most proximal part.

INSERTION

The insertion of a muscle is normally the most movable point of attachment, and is its most distal part.

Origin and insertion reversed. Muscles act on joints and usually move the joint nearest to the insertion first, and then in continued action will move the next joint over which the muscle passes, if any. However muscles can move the joint nearest to their point of origin first and this is called origin and insertion reversed. For example, sitting up, using the abdominal muscles, is an example of origin and insertion reversed.

ATTACHMENT

The attachment of muscles can be by muscle fibres, tendons, or fibrous bands called aponeurosis, to each other, bones, skin, ligaments, fascia, or cartilage.

SHAPE

The shape of the muscles depends upon how they run from their origin to their insertion, and the arrangement of the muscle fibres within this direction. Sometimes the muscles run directly and straight down from one point of attachment to the other, and sometimes they run obliquely from the origin to the insertion.

Fibres of straight running muscles can be *quadrilateral, fusiform,* or *straplike* (Figure 11). All these shaped muscles give great range of movement and speed.

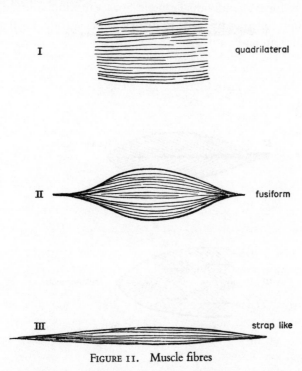

I   quadrilateral

II   fusiform

III   strap like

FIGURE 11.   Muscle fibres

Fibres of obliquely running muscles usually have a central tendon with short fibres going into it (Figure 12). They can be *unipennate,* with the fibres directed to one side only of the tendon, *bi-pennate* with the fibres lying on either side of the central tendon, or *multi-pennate* where there are several small tendons into which the fibres converge. These shaped muscles are designed for power of movement.

CONTRACTION

The contraction of muscle depends upon the shortening in length of the muscle fibres. The muscle fibres contract up to forty per cent. However, even when a muscle appears to be tightly contracted, some of its fibres are relaxed. These remain at the ready to take over, relieving those that are working at full capacity, throughout the contraction.

I   unipennate

II   bipennate

III   multi-pennate

FIGURE 12.   Muscle fibres

TONE

The tone of muscle is that degree of slight constant contraction which remains in the muscle fibres of the most relaxed muscles. Those muscle fibres which are not in a state of slight tension periodically take over from those that are, to avoid strain and fatigue, when the muscle appears to be at rest.

ACTION

The action of muscle is upon the joints, and when any particular movement takes place, several muscles or groups of muscles are brought into action to perform a specific function in a combined effort. These muscles are called protagonists, antagonists, fixators, and synergists.

Protagonists are the prime movers in any muscle action, that is, the contracting muscle which produces the main action required.

Antagonists are the controlling influence upon the prime movers. They are usually the muscles which perform the opposite movement to that required and their function is to relax whilst the protagonists contract.

Fixators are the stabilizers of the movement. They work to fix, hold, and steady the bones either at the origin or insertion part from which the prime movers come. They cut out unnecessary movement produced elsewhere which would hinder the prime movers.

Synergists also prevent inefficiency and help the protagonists to produce the best possible movements. They fix the joints which are not required to move but over which the prime movers pass, and therefore would have to move if it were not for the synergists. By their action they place the joints not required to move in a position which ensures maximum power and efficiency for the protagnoists, e.g. making a fist requires the wrist to be extended and held in this position, the flexors of the wrist then only flex tightly the fingers and thumb.

The action of individual muscles is very difficult to define for they work together in groups and the groups come into action as a team. There may be one or more muscles involved in producing an action as a protagonist and also several muscles involved in the rest of the team work, as antagonists, fixators, and synergists. However, although the individual muscle can be said to have one main action, most muscles are capable of producing several other actions. The muscle deltoid is a multi-pennate muscle, with middle, anterior, and posterior fibres. Its action as a whole produces abduction of the arm, but its anterior fibres may contract to help flex the arm and its posterior fibres can contract to extend the arm. Sometimes gravity can affect and alter the muscle groups which are brought into play during a specific movement. For example, in flexion of the trunk from the standing position, it is the flexor muscles of the trunk which start the movement. As gravity exerts its pull the back extensors take over. However, it can be seen that it is only the co-ordination of all the muscle groups together which will produce a smooth efficient performance.

NERVES

The nerves of the muscle cause the muscle to contract and convey messages to the brain which are essential for co-ordination and positioning. The brain only registers patterns of movements and not muscle contractions. It is only when the action of a muscle is known that it can be made to contract.

BLOOD SUPPLY

Blood supply to the muscles is rich and abundant.

TENDONS AND APONEUROSIS

Tendons and aponeurosis are the structures which connect the muscles to the bones. A tendon is a tough, fibrous, inelastic, cord-like end of a muscle sometimes called a girder or sinew. It is sometimes surrounded by a synovial sheath which serves to prevent friction by secreting synovial fluid which in turn acts as a lubricant in the same way as for the joints. Sometimes the synovial membrane of these sheaths becomes inflamed due to strain as in 'teno-synovitis' at the wrist, when the tendons become swollen and movement is very painful. Bursae may also be present in between the tendon and bone again preventing friction. An aponeurosis is a flattened-out tendon. Both have a poor blood supply. Tendons require special attention in massage, such as finger kneadings and frictions, to stimulate the blood supply.

FASCIA

Fascia of the body is a membrane of variable thickness which runs throughout the body. It is divided into two layers, a superficial and deep layer.

Superficial fascia lies directly beneath the skin over the whole body. It consists of areolar connective tissue permeated with fat. The thickness varies in different parts of the body. Women are more evenly supplied than men, and because this fatty layer is thicker in women, their contours are softer and rounder than men. It acts as a protection, and fat being a bad conductor of heat helps to prevent heat loss from the body, so that it helps to keep the body warm. It enables the skin to move easily because of its elasticity and mobility. Shielding underlying structures, it allows blood vessels and nerves to split up into it before continuing their final destination into the skin. In the palms of the hands, feet, and in the scalp, it is tougher and more fibrous, binding down the skin to the structures beneath it. It is absent in areas such as the eyelids but abundant in the abdominal area, so this area tends to accumulate an envelope of fat. Certain muscles insert directly into the superficial fascia, e.g. platysma muscle.

Deep fascia lies below the superficial fascia and consists of tough inelastic fibrous membrane, binding and ensheathing muscles and muscle groups together. The muscles can contract against this strong band of tissue and sometimes originate and insert into it. In areas like the ankles and wrists the deep fascia can form thickened tunnels, separating and binding the tendons to the bone, preventing them from splaying out. In other areas it sends off fibrous partitions which dip between the muscles and separate them, blending with the periosteum. The deep fascia also surrounds the blood vessels and nerves providing them with fascial pathways to their terminations.

[Muscles of the Shoulder

Muscles of the Shoulder

NAME	ORIGIN	INSERTION	ACTION
Deltoid Gives the rounded shape of the shoulder. Triangular-shaped muscle. Three sets of fibres	Spine of scapula acromion process. Outer third clavicle	Deltoid tuberosity on upper third of humerus	Abduction of arm, anterior fibres flex arm, posterior extend arm
Supra-spinatus When the muscle is sprained abduction of the arm is poor	Supra-spinous fossa on scapula	Great tuberosity of humerus	Fixes head of humerus whilst deltoid works
Infra spinatus Works with teres minor	Infra-spinous fossa on scapula	Great tuberosity of humerus	Outwardly rotates the arm

Teres major	Dorsum of lateral border of scapula	Bicipital groove on humerus	Inwardly rotates, adducts, and extends arm
Teres minor	Dorsum of lateral border of scapula	Great tuberosity of humerus	Laterally rotates arm
Subscapularis Works with latissimus dorsi	Anterior aspect of scapula	Lesser tuberosity of humerus	Medially rotates arm
Coraco–brachialis	Coracoid process	Middle of medial surface of humerus	Flexes arm, helps to adduct arm

Muscles of the Upper Arm

See Figure 13.

NAME	ORIGIN	INSERTION	ACTION
Biceps Lies on front of arm, two heads	Supra-glenoid tuberosity on scapula. Coracoid process	Radial tuberosity on radius	Supinates forearm, flexes forearm, helps to fix head of humerus
Triceps Has three heads, lies on back of arm	Scapula and capsule of shoulder joint. Upper half humerus. Lower half humerus.	Olecranon process of ulna	Extends the forearm
Brachialis Lies below biceps	Lower half humerus	Ulna	Flexes the forearm

Back view

Front view

deltoid

triceps

brachioradialis

extensor carpi
radialis longus

anconeus

extensors

flexor
carpi
ulnaris

abductor pollicis
longus

extensor pollicis
brevis

extensor pollicis
longus

biceps

triceps

brachialis

pronator
teres

flexor carpi
radialis

flexor digitorum
sublimis

flexor carpi
ulnaris

palmaris longus

thenar
muscles

palmaris brevis

hypothenar
eminence

FIGURE 13. Muscles of the right arm

Muscles of Forearm and Hand

The muscles on the forearm can be divided into two groups: the anterior flexor group and the posterior extensor group of muscles. These in turn are divided into a superficial group and a deep group.

SUPERFICIAL FLEXOR GROUP

This group consists of several muscles which originate from the medial epicondyle of the humerus and from a common flexor tendon.

NAME	ORIGIN	INSERTION	ACTION
Pronatorteres Crosses the forearm obliquely	Common flexor tendon	Lower shaft of radius	Pronates forearm turning palm of hand backwards
Palmaris longus	Common flexor tendon	Palmar fascia	Flexes hand
Flexor carpi radialis	Common flexor tendon	Second and third metacarpal bones	Flexes and abducts hand

NAME	ORIGIN	INSERTION	ACTION
Flexor carpi ulnaris	Common flexor tendon, and ulna	Carpals, and fifth metacarpal	Flexes and adducts hand
Flexor digitorum sublimis	Common flexor tendon, ulna, and radius	Divides into four tendons inserting into middle phalanges	Flexes fingers and then wrist

DEEP FLEXOR GROUP

This group consists of muscles which lie underneath the superficial layer on the anterior surface of the forearm.

NAME	ORIGIN	INSERTION	ACTION
Pronator quadratus	Lower third of ulna	Lower third of radius	Pronates the forearm. Hand turns backwards
Flexor pollicis longus	Middle of radius and ulna	Distal phalanx of thumb	Flexes thumb
Flexor digitorum profundus	Ulna and interosseous membrane	Divides into four tendons inserting into distal phalanges	Flexes fingers and wrist

Muscles of Forearm and Hand continued

SUPERFICIAL EXTENSOR GROUP

These consist of muscles which lie on the posterior and lateral side of the forearm and arise from a common tendon originating from the lateral epicondyle of the humerus.

NAME	ORIGIN	INSERTION	ACTION
Brachioradialis Most superficial of all the muscles	Humerus	Radius, styloid process	Flexes elbow joint
Extensor carpi radialis longus	Common extensor tendon, and humerus	Third metacarpal	Extends and abducts hand
Extensor carpi radialis brevis	Common extensor tendon	Third metacarpal	Extends and abducts hand
Extensor digitorum	Common extensor tendon	Proximal phalanx of little finger	Extends the fingers
Extensor digiti minimi	Common extensor tendon	Fifth metacarpal	Extends little finger
Anconeus Assists the work of triceps, is a small triangular-shaped muscle on back of elbow joint	Lower lateral side of humerus	Olecranon process of ulna	Extends forearm at elbow joint

DEEP EXTENSOR GROUP

These muscles all lie underneath the superficial group and cross over from the back of the forearm to the radial side.

NAME	ORIGIN	INSERTION	ACTION
Supinator	Lateral epicondyle of humerus, and ulna	Surrounds upper third of radius	Supinates forearm
Abductor pollicis longus	Ulna and radius	First metacarpal	Abducts thumb
Extensor pollicis brevis	Radius, and interosseous membrane	Proximal phalanx of thumb	Extends proximal phalanx of thumb
Extensor pollicis longus	Ulna and interosseous membrane	Distal phalanx of thumb	Extends distal phalanx
Extensor indicis Lies below extensor pollicis longus	Ulna and interosseous membrane	Second metacarpal	Extends index finger at metacarpo-phalangeal joint, and wrist

Muscles of the Hand

The muscles of the hand can be divided into three groups: the thenar eminence, which lies laterally and is the fleshy ball of the thumb; the hypothenar eminence, which is the small medial fleshy mass of the little finger; and the muscles which lie in between the metacarpal bones of the hand and palm. All these muscles are concerned with the fine movements of the fingers.

The small muscle of the thumb which draws the thumb across the palm is called the *opponens pollicis*. The other muscles of the thumb are *flexor pollicis brevis, abductor pollicis brevis*, and *adductor pollicis brevis*. They all arise from one or more of the carpal bones nearest the thumb and from the metacarpal bones. They are inserted into the phalanges or metacarpal bone of the thumb. Their actions are restricted purely to fine movements of the thumb as their name suggests, without which the hand would be almost useless. They flex, abduct, and adduct the thumb.

Muscles of the little finger are all called digiti minimi. These muscles originate mainly from the medial carpal bones and insert into the metacarpal or proximal phalanx of the little fingers. They in turn act on the little fingers helping to flex and draw them medially so deepening the palm.

Muscles which lie between the bones are called the *lumbrical* and *interossei* muscles. They arise from the tendons of flexor digitorum profundus in the middle of the palm and insert into the extensor tendons on the phalanges. These muscles help to flex the metacarpo-phalangeal joint and extend the middle and distal phalanges at the same time. The interossei muscles are attached to the metacarpal bones, and fill in the spaces between these bones. They perform the action of abduction and adduction (separating and closing) of the fingers together with extending the proximal and distal interphalangeal joints.

The index finger and thumb have their own abductors and the thumb has an adductor, therefore no interossei muscles are inserted into the bones of these digits, and only one interossei which adducts is supplied to the little finger. The interossei which adduct are called the palmar interossei, and those which abduct are called the dorsal interossei because of their attachments.

Muscles of Buttocks and Thigh

In the buttock region the tissues are unusually dense and thick, because the superficial fascia in this area is exceptionally fatty, being more common in women than in men, and also because the large prominence, of the buttock, which is one of the most characteristic features of Man's muscular system, is composed of a coarse broad fleshy mass of muscle ensheathed in fascia called *gluteus maximus*. This muscle performs an enormous task, which is that of keeping the body upright, so that by virtue of its very function it has to be strong, tough, and unyielding. Normally, in the upright standing position, the gluteal muscles help to maintain an erect posture by working in co-ordination with the flexor muscles of the hip. When the gluteal muscles work origin and insertion reversed, they can extend the trunk on the thigh, with the hamstrings. The gluteus medius and minimus are responsible for correct balance when walking. As the leg is raised on one side the muscles tilt the pelvis slightly on that side, but at the same time they pull it downwards to the supporting leg side so that the body does not topple. The deep gluteal fascia of the buttocks and thigh is called the *fascia lata*. Some of this fascia separates the muscles of the thigh into an anterior and posterior compartment. The ilio-tibial band or tract is another feature of the deep fascia in this area helping to steady the femur on the tibia. It lies on the lateral aspect of the thigh being attached above to the iliac crest and below to the lateral tibial condyle covering the tensor fascia femoris muscle completely.

[Gluteal Muscles

Gluteal Muscles

NAME	ORIGIN	INSERTION	ACTION
Gluteus maximus Most superficial and largest muscle	Iliac crest, sacral fascia	Gluteal ridge below great trochanter, ilio-tibial tract	Extension of thigh, lateral rotation of thigh, and hip joint
Gluteus medius Lies partly beneath gluteus maximus	Ilium (crest)	Great trochanter	Abduction of thigh, medially rotates thigh
Gluteus minimus Lies beneath gluteus medius and is deepest of all gluteal muscles	Ilium (crest)	Great trochanter	Abducts thigh, medially rotates thigh
Tensor fasciae femoris Situated anteriorly and laterally on the thigh	Ilium, (anterior superior spine)	Into fascia lata below great trochanter	Abducts thigh, inwardly rotates thigh

Piriformis, obturator internus, and externus, gemellus superior and inferior, and quadratus femoris are all muscles deeply placed in the gluteal and hip region. Their action is to rotate the thigh outwards.

Quadriceps Muscles on Front of Thigh

See Figure 14.

NAME	ORIGIN	INSERTION	ACTION
Rectus femoris			
Most superficial muscle	Front of ilium, on anterior inferior spine, acetabulum	Patella	Extension of leg on thigh at knee joint, flexion of thigh at hip joint
Vastus lateralis	Femur (great trochanter area)	Patella, tibial tubercle	Extension of knee joint
Vastus medialis	Femur (great trochanter area)	Patella, tibial tubercle	Extension of knee joint
Vastus intermedius			
Deepest of quadriceps	Upper two thirds of shaft of femur	Patella, tibial tubercle	Extension of knee joint

FIGURE 14.   Muscles of the right leg

Other Muscles Acting on Thigh

Iliacus and psoas arise from the ilium and are inserted into the top of the femur. They are very powerful hip flexors, flexing the thigh on the pelvis.

Articularis genu lies below the quadriceps and helps to extend the knee.

Pectineus arises from the pubis and is inserted into the femur. It adducts and flexes the thigh.

Sartorius is a superficial long thin strap-like muscle extending from the anterior iliac spine crossing the front of the thigh to the medial side of the tibia. It flexes and medially rotates the leg on the thigh, and also flexes the thigh on the pelvis abducts and outwardly rotates the thigh.

Femoral Triangle

The femoral triangle is an area situated on the upper and medial aspect of the thigh. When the thigh is flexed, abducted, and outwardly rotated, as in the cross-legged sitting position, it can be seen quite clearly as a triangular depression. A ligament forms its base and its boundaries are formed by the adductor longus medially, and the sartorius muscle laterally. In this area lie nerves, arteries, veins, and the important inguinal lymph glands draining the lymphatic vessels of the lower limb.

[Adductor Muscles on Medial Side of Thigh

Adductor Muscles on Medial Side of Thigh

NAME	ORIGIN	INSERTION	ACTION
Adductor magnus Situated on inner side of thigh deepest of adductor muscles, three sets of fibres	Ischial tuberosity, ischium, pubis	Inner shaft of femur	Adducts thigh, flexes thigh. Extends thigh, outwardly rotates thigh
Adductor longus Superficial muscle of adductor muscles on inner side of thigh	Pubis (tendonous)	Middle shaft of femur	Adduction, outward rotation and flexion of thigh
Adductor brevis Situated on the inner and upper part of the thigh	Pubis (aponeurosis)	Upper shaft of femur	Adduction, outward rotation and flexion of thigh
Gracilis Situated near the surface on the inner side of the thigh	Ischium pubis	Upper part of shaft of tibia	Inward rotation of leg and flexion. Adduction of thigh and flexion of thigh in hip

Hamstring Muscles on Back of Thigh

The hamstrings help to raise the trunk upright from the stooping position. They bend the knee.

NAME	ORIGIN	INSERTION	ACTION
Biceps femoris Two heads	Ischial tuberosity femur	Head of fibula	Flexes the leg at knee joint, rotates leg laterally. Extends thigh at hip joint
Semimembranosus	Ischial tuberosity (thick tendon)	Medial condyle of tibia	Flexes leg and medially rotates leg
Semitendinosus	Ischial tuberosity	Medial condyle of tibia	Flexes leg on thigh and medially rotates it

Muscles of the Lower Leg

These muscles can be divided into three groups: those on the front, those on the anterior and lateral side, and those on the medial and posterior side of the leg.

FRONT OF LEG

NAME	ORIGIN	INSERTION	ACTION
Tibialis anterior Superficial muscle on front of leg. Tendon crosses over front of ankle, lying innermost	Upper two thirds of tibia	Medial cuneiform first metatarsal	Dorsiflexes foot, inverts foot
Extensor digitorum longus Superficial muscle	Tibia, upper two thirds of fibula anteriorly, interosseous membrane	Split tendon into middle and distal phalanges of second, third, fourth and fifth toes	Extension of metatarsal-phalangeal joint, of four outer toes. Dorsiflexion of ankle joint
Extensor hallucis longus Lies deep to extensor digitorum longus	Lower two thirds of fibula	Distal phalanx of big toe	Extends metatarsal-phalangeal joint of big toe
Peroneus tertius	Lower lateral	Fifth metatarsal	Dorsiflexes foot,

ANTERIOR AND LATERAL SIDE OF LEG

NAME	ORIGIN	INSERTION	ACTION
Peroneus longus Most superficial on lateral aspect of leg. Lies on outer side of leg, and sole of the foot	Upper two thirds of fibula	Medial cuneiform	Plantar flexes foot, everts foot
Peroneus brevis Lies beneath peroneus longus	Lower two thirds of fibula	Base of fifth metatarsal	Plantar flexes foot, everts foot

CALF MUSCLES ON MEDIAL AND POSTERIOR SIDE OF LEG
SUPERFICIAL GROUP

NAME	ORIGIN	INSERTION	ACTION
Gastrocnemius Most superficial providing bulk of the calf	Condyles of femur (two heads)	Calcaneum (by tendo achilles)	Plantar flexes foot, provides the push forwards in walking and running

B.M.—6*

Calf Muscles continued

NAME	ORIGIN	INSERTION	ACTION
Soleus	Fibula and tibia	Calcaneum	Helps gastrocnemius
Plantaris	Lateral condyle of femur	Calcaneum	Helps gastrocnemius
	DEEP GROUP		
Popliteus Flat triangular muscle	Lateral condyle of femur	Shaft of tibia	Flexes knee joint, rotates lower leg medially
Flexor hallucis longus	Middle of fibula	Distal phalanx of big toe	Flexes big toe
Flexor digitorum longus Deep to back of leg on the inner side	Middle of tibia	Four tendons of distal phalanx of outer four toes	Flexes toes, plantar flexes ankle
Tibialis posterior Deep on posterior aspect of leg	Fibula, tibia, interosseous membrane	Talus, navicular three cuneiforms, second and third metatarsal	Inverts foot, plantar flexes foot

Muscles on Sole of the Foot

There are four layers of short muscles situated on the plantar aspect of the foot. They originate mainly from the tarsal bones, ligaments, and tendons of the long muscles but, as each layer deepens into the sole, their origins move forwards progressively. Their function and action is to maintain the arches of the foot which are formed by the design and shape of the bones, and to propel and push the body forwards in walking.

FIRST LAYER

Abductor hallucis: abducts the big toe.

Flexor digitorum brevis: flexes the toes.

Abductor digiti minimi: abducts the little toe.

SECOND LAYER

Flexor digitorum accessorius: aids flexion of all the toes.

Lumbricals: aids extension of the toes.

THIRD LAYER

Flexor hallucis brevis: flexes the big toe.

Adductor hallucis obliqus and transversus: adducts the big toe and raises the metatarsal arch.

Flexor digiti minimi brevis: flexes the little toe.

FOURTH LAYER

Interossei: extend the toes, and flex the metatarso-phalangeal joint. There are four dorsal interossei which abduct the toes, and three plantar interossei which adduct the toes.

Muscle on Dorsum of the Foot

Extensor digitorum brevis is the only short muscle on this aspect of the foot. It is a thin muscle and its action is to extend the outer four toes to all the phalangeal joints but only to extend the first phalanx of the big toe into which it is inserted. This muscle does not exist in the corresponding hand and is essential in the foot to give the big toe an extra push when walking.

Popliteal fossa is the area behind the knee which contains nerves, veins, arteries, and lymph glands. It can be seen clearly if the knee is slightly flexed against a resistance. The floor of this space is formed by the muscle popliteus from which the name is derived.

Tendo-Achilles is the name given to the tendon of the gastrocnemius muscle which together with the soleus and plantaris is inserted into the calcaneum. The heel of the mythical Greek hero Achilles was his only vulnerable spot. He was shot in it by an arrow from one of his enemies, and died. Thus the common usage of the expression 'Achilles heel' is taken to mean vulnerability, but in anatomy refers to the above-mentioned tendon.

Muscles on the Back of the Trunk

There are three superficial layers of back muscles (Figure 15). The first two superficial layers connect the upper limb and shoulder girdle to the trunk. All the muscles of the back, including the third and deepest layer, are concerned with extension of the spine and play an important role in keeping the body upright, raising it from the bending position.

FIRST LAYER

The first layer, and most superficial, consists of the muscles trapezius and latissimus dorsi. Trapezius stretches from the base of the thorax to the occiput and out to the peak of the shoulder. One on its own is triangular in shape but both sides together are trapezoid. Latissimus dorsi is situated in the lower half of the back and spine and the upper part of the arm. It helps to form the posterior wall of the axilla.

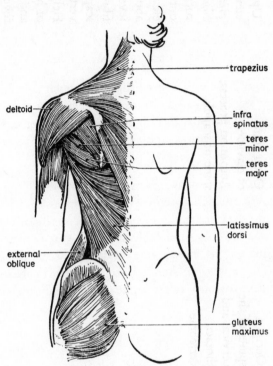

FIGURE 15.   Muscles of the back

Back Muscles

FIRST LAYER

NAME	ORIGIN	INSERTION	ACTION
Trapezius	Occiput, spines of the cervical and thoracic vertebrae	Outer third of clavicle. Acromion process, spine of scapula	Upper fibres elevate shoulder girdle. All fibres working rotate scapula outwards to elevate arm above shoulder level. Middle fibres adduct scapula towards vertebral column. Helps extension of head origin and insertion reversed
Latissimus dorsi Fibres are directed upwards and outwards.	Spines of lower thoracic vertebrae,	Bicipital groove on humerus	Adducts the arm. Inward rotation

Its tendon twists upon itself	lumbar fascia, spines of lumbar vertebrae, iliac crest, lower four ribs, inferior angle of scapula		of arm, and extension of arm. Raises body towards the arm when origin and insertion are reversed, as in climbing

SECOND LAYER

Levator scapuli Situated at the back of the neck from the vertebral column to the superior angle of scapula. Fibres are directed downwards and outwards	Upper four cervical vertebrae	Medial border of scapula between spine and superior angle	Rotates inferior angle of scapula inwards. Both muscles working elevates shoulder girdle. Origin and insertion reversed extends cervical spine. (Braces back shoulder girdle)

Back Muscles continued

NAME	ORIGIN	INSERTION	ACTION
Rhomboid minor Situated between spinal column and scapula	Spines of seventh cervical and first thoracic vertebrae	Medial border of scapula opposite root of spine	Adducts scapula towards vertebral column. Inwardly rotates inferior angle of scapula. (Braces back shoulder girdle)
Rhomboid major Situated between spinal column, and scapula below rhomboid minor	Second, third, and fourth thoracic spine and ligaments	Medial border of scapula below spine	Adducts scapula towards spine bracing shoulder girdle backwards

THIRD LAYER

This deep layer of back muscles consists of *splenius capitus* and *splenius cervicus* which lie deep in the neck of the trapezius and extend the neck when both sides work, rotating it to the same side when only one side works. Also in this layer of muscles is *serratus posterior superior* situated at the base of the neck and upper part of the thorax, and it rotates the trunk to the opposite side as well as acting on the ribs. The *serratus posterior inferior* is situated in the upper lumbar and lower thoracic region and rotates the trunk to the opposite side as well as acting on the ribs.

DEEP LAYER OF BACK MUSCLES

The erector spinae muscles of the back lie in the deepest layer of the back muscles. The beauty therapist should note that finger frictions and kneadings are applied either side of the spine particularly for this muscle. This muscle originates from the posterior surface of the sacrum, the iliac crest, and from the spines of the lumbar vertebrae. It passes upwards attaching to the transverse processes of the vertebrae and inserts into the base of the occiput and mastoid process. As this muscle extends upwards it divides into three groups sending slips out to be attached to the ribs. It helps to extend the spine with the other deep muscles of the back, which do not unduly concern the beauty therapist.

Muscles of Neck and Chest

The muscles which are of important interest to the beauty therapist in this region are the sterno-mastoid, platysma, the pectoral muscles, and serratus anterior (Figure 16).

Diaphragm muscle is the muscle which separates the thorax from the abdomen. It is a large dome-shaped muscle originating from the sternum, the lower six ribs, and the upper lumbar vertebrae. It is inserted into a strong central tendon at the peak of its dome. This muscle is the chief muscle of respiration. When it contracts on inspiration the pressures inside the thorax and abdomen are

FIGURE 16. Muscles of the trunk (right side)

altered. On inspiration the rib cage expands and the abdominal organs descend. On expiration the diaphragm relaxes, the abdominal contents ascend, and, as the rib cage collapses, air is forced out of the lungs. The diaphragm plays an important part in labour, together with the abdominal muscles, when it helps to expel the baby out of the birth canal, by pushing downwards.

NECK MUSCLES

NAME	ORIGIN	INSERTION	ACTION
Platysma	Fascia on front of chest	Mandible below chin blending with fibres of muscle on opposite side	Depresses the lower jaw
Sterno–mastoid	By two heads from sternum and clavicle	Occiput temporal bone	Both together flex the head. One rotates the head to the opposite side, and side flexes the head to the same side

CHEST MUSCLES

NAME	ORIGIN	INSERTION	ACTION
Pectoralis major	Clavicle, sternum, upper six ribs	Bicipital groove of humerus	Adducts the arm, flexes the arm with deltoid

CHEST MUSCLES—*continued*

NAME	ORIGIN	INSERTION	ACTION
Pectoralis minor Lies under pectoralis major	Third and fourth ribs	Coracoid process of scapula	Pulls scapula downwards and forwards
Serratus Anterior When the shoulder blade protrudes abnormally in a condition called 'winged scapula' it is because this muscle is either paralysed or very weak	Upper eight ribs (side of chest wall)	Vertebral (Medial) border of scapula	Pulls the scapula onto the ribs. When the arm is raised to shoulder level it helps to rotate the scapula, and elevate the arm. It is the force in the punching action of the arms

Axilla

The axilla (armpit) is the large hollow depression found underneath the top of the arm. It houses important lymph glands, arteries, veins, and nerves.

Muscles of the Abdominal Wall

NAME	ORIGIN	INSERTION	ACTION
Rectus abdominis	Pubic crest	Sternum and lower ribs	Flexes spine and aids respiration. Helps in lifting legs upwards on trunk
External oblique	Lower eight ribs	Iliac crest	When one muscle works bends trunk to opposite side, and side flexes to same side. Flexes trunk when both work
Internal oblique	Iliac crest, lumbar fascia	Lower six ribs, rectus abdominis fascia	Bends trunk to same side, and side flexes trunk to same side, when one muscle works. Flexes trunk when both work together

Muscles of the Abdominal Wall continued

NAME	ORIGIN	INSERTION	ACTION
Transversalis	Iliac crest, lumbar fascia, lower six ribs	Xiphoid process, fascia between umbilicus, and pubis	Aids outer abdominal muscles in all their actions, and functions
Quadratus lumborum Is the muscle on the back of the abdomen situated in the back of the waist	Iliac crest	Last rib, upper four lumbar vertebrae	Side flexes the trunk in the lumbar region, to the same side. Extends lumbar vertebrae

Muscles of Scalp and Facial Expression

The scalp consists of several layers. Its outermost covering of the skin is tough and thick. The next layer consists of blood vessels and nerves and the tendons of two muscles frontalis and occipitalis from the third layer running over the scalp and forehead. It is then connected to a loose layer of tissue which facilitates movement over the cranium especially when massaging. The final layer is the equivalent to the periosteum on the bones of the body, and is called the pericranium.

The facial expression muscles have very little attachment to bone, and they are all inserted into the skin producing the various expressions. *See* Figure 17.

FIGURE 17. Muscles of the face

NAMES AND ACTIONS OF MUSCLES OF EXPRESSION

Scalp and forehead: Occipito frontalis pulls scalp backwards and produces transverse lines of forehead.

Eyelids: Orbicularis oculi closes eyes gently and tightly, *corrugator* produces the vertical frown, *levator palpebrae superioris* raises eyelids.

Ear: Auricularis twitches ear.

Nose: Procerus wrinkles bridge of nose, *compressor naris* compresses the nostrils, *depressor septi* widens nostrils, *dilator naris* dilates the nostrils.

Mouth: Orbicularis oris surrounds mouth, squeezes mouth tightly together, *levator labii* lifts upper lip, *levator anguli oris* lifts corner of mouth upwards, *zygomaticus* lifts mouth and cheeks upwards in laughing, *depressor labii inferioris* turns lower lip down, *mentalis* wrinkles chin and makes lower lip protrude, *platysma* is muscle over lower jaw and neck, *buccinator* blows out cheeks, *risorius* produces grinning.

9. *Passive Movements*

Passive movements are those movements given to the client which are performed by the beauty therapist alone and in which the client plays no active part. They can be divided into two groups, forced and relaxed. Forced passive movements are mainly carried out under medical supervision. It is only the relaxed passive movements which concern the beauty therapist and which will be described. They may be given as a treatment on their own, included as a part of the massage session or merely used as a method of handling the client's limbs whilst re-positioning during the course of treatment.

POINTS OF IMPORTANCE

As in massage the client must be warm and comfortable. The position of the therapist is important because she must be able to move the joints of the client easily and effortlessly. She should as in massage, face the client at all times and be aware of any untoward expression that would indicate a temporary cessation or modification of treatment. The handling of the client's limbs must be firm enough to instil a feeling of complete confidence in the client, but care must be taken not to nip or squeeze too tightly with the hand grips, as this will be painful and cause tension. Once having mastered the technique of holding, grasping, and moving the joints and limbs, the same methods should be utilized and applied when merely moving a part of the body to another position. Apart from the sense of confidence and security the client feels in the therapist and treatment if her limbs are moved firmly, stress and strain on the joints, ligaments, and tendons is avoided when the limbs are adequately supported. There is nothing more irritating and less inspiring than handling a client as though she were a wet fish, being pushed, prodded, and plonked into position. It is important to localize the movements to the joint being moved, by immobilizing the other joints above and below. Traction or a gentle pull in the long direction of the bones separating their joint surfaces is advisable to ensure a perfectly free movement. Slight overpressure at the completion of flexion, and a little extra stretching at the end of extension help to guarantee full range of movement. If the client is very tense it may take several treatments before the maximum movement possible is obtained. Forcing a movement can cause muscle spasm and tension which will restrict the movement, so defeating the object of relaxed passive movements. Sometimes it may help a client before giving the treatment if the therapist demonstrates on herself first the type of movements that are required.

CONTRA-INDICATIONS

Contra-indications of passive movements would be when there are conditions present which require medical treatment. If pain is experienced on passive movements then they should be discontinued in that joint. Some chronic arthritic conditions of joints are improved by passive movements providing that the movements are only taken to the limit that the condition imposes. Where joints are hot and swollen, or the skin around them shiny, the movements are not advisable. If passive movements are properly administered there is no danger of damaging the soft structures of the joints, and therefore very few contra-indications.

EFFECTS AND USES

1. Relaxation is the main effect of these kind of movements. Passive movements if performed smoothly, slowly, and rhythmically without any break in continuity have a soothing

effect. A tense client can be taught to relax the whole body or any localized area.

2. Passive movements to the head can deplete the flow of blood to the head, tension in the cranial muscles is also relaxed, and tension headaches can be soothed. Strain and anxiety which soon shows on the face will be reduced.

3. Suppleness in the joints can be improved through passive movements, and this may be shown by more graceful and fluid movements in everyday functional activity.

4. Stiffness due to insufficient exercise or over-exercising may be removed by gradually increasing the range of movement, aches and pains being eased away. This in turn will give rise to a more pleasant facial expression and will relieve tension elsewhere, improving all-round general posture.

5. They may be given as a preliminary to massage to assess the type of client in order to find out whether she is tense or relaxed, and if there is any limitation of movement in the joints. The treatment can then be tailored if necessary to suit the individual requirements of the client.

6. The hand grips and support of the joints and limbs which are used in passive movements can be conveniently applied when lifting the limbs from one position to another during the course of other treatments.

7. Passive movements may encourage and prepare a client for more active exercises on her own.

8. In the joints moved, the synovial fluid is increased and therefore the joints are fed, nourished, and lubricated. Waste products are absorbed and removed, adhesions prevented, and the mobility of the joints, if not increased, is certainly maintained independently of muscular activity.

9. Muscle tone can be decreased in the muscles which pass over the joint being moved. In cases where they are shortened and tight they could be gradually eased into a state of relaxation and gently stretched. This would improve the range of movement in the joint without force although it may take several regular treatments to accomplish. The effect would be, depending upon which muscle groups are contracted, to

improve the posture and carriage of the client. For instance, tight pectoral muscles can lead to round shoulders; hip flexors, or tightened hamstrings, could restrict mobility of the spine again causing a defective picture. This leads to compensatory stress and strain on other parts of the body which eventually might need medical attention.

10. Venous circulation is aided as the veins passing over the joints are squeezed and stretched by the rhythmic smooth movements. This can help warm up different areas and improve the cosmetic appearance of cold blue limbs due to sluggish circulation. The movements must be done quickly and vigorously. Circumduction of the shoulder and hip joints would be most effective in these cases. Circumduction of the hip joint will also increase the flow of blood to the abdomen, relieving abdominal stasis and aiding digestion.

11. Extensibility of the muscles passing over the joints can be increased as relaxation in them improves, although muscle tone is not effected with passive movements.

12. Sometimes passive movements are given for their stimulating effect. They could be given as a full treatment to a lethargic, tired client, or to clients who have neither time nor energy for active exercises. Although they cannot replace active exercise, they do ensure that the joints and muscles are moved through their full range. Very few people use their muscles and joints to their full limit in every-day functional activity. With a stimulating treatment of passive movements, the joint and muscle sense is stimulated, and there is a reflex contraction in the opposing muscle group of each movement; the brain becomes aware of the movement. As the nerves, arteries, and veins pass over the joints they are alternately stretched and compressed. Speeding up the activity of these vessels invokes a general feeling of alertness. The movements here would be done quickly and briskly, maintaining a good rhythm, but with a more staccato pattern of movement than employed when giving passive movements for their soothing effect. With the emphasis on physical stimulation by passive movements, the way could be paved for more active

exercises, and the client should feel refreshed, invigorated, and raring to go.

13. Leaving the client with a sense of being thoroughly and completely treated is another effect of passive movements in beauty therapy if one or two movements are given to each joint during or after the course of a massage treatment.

Technique

MOVEMENTS AND GRIPS IN LYING

RIGHT ARM

Shoulder joint: The client can be lying near the edge of the couch or in sitting with the therapist in stride standing beside her. The client's elbow must be slightly flexed with the hand pronated. Grasping the client's elbow firmly with her left hand, the therapist holds the client's right hand and wrist in the thumb and finger grip. This involves placing the index and middle fingers round the client's thumb and palm, with the thumb, fourth, and fifth fingers of the therapist firmly encircling the wrist to prevent movement in this joint. During all the movements of the shoulder joint the therapist's left hand pivots round the point of the elbow and the utmost care must be taken to see that full weight of the limb is borne by the therapist.

Order of Movements

1. Circumduction to mobilize the joint.
2. Flexion into elevation.
3. Extension from elevation through flexion.
4. Abduction into elevation.
5. Adduction from elevation through abduction.
6. Inward rotation.
7. Outward rotation.
8. Circumduction.

Elbow joint: The beauty therapist is in walk standing with the client in the same position as for the shoulder joint. Keeping the same thumb and finger grip, the therapist's left hand slides to support the elbow from the back and just above it. The hand is supinated.

Order of movements

1. Flexion.
2. Extension.
3. Pronation to the forearm with the elbow semi-flexed.
4. Supination with the elbow semi-flexed.

Wrist joint: The position of the client and therapist remains unchanged, except that the upper arm is supported to the elbow, which is semi-flexed, with the hand in pronation. The beauty therapist firmly holds the forearm just above the wrist joint with her left hand, modifying the thumb and finger grip, by retracting her thumb and outer two fingers to below the client's wrist, leaving it completely free.

Order of movements

1. Circumduction for mobility.
2. Flexion.
3. Extension.
4. Abduction (radial deviation).
5. Adduction (ulnar deviation).
6. Circumduction.

Metacarpo-phalangeal joints: The therapist places the fingers of her left hand across the palm of the hand above the joints with her thumb across the dorsal aspect of the client's hand to isolate the movements to these joints. Each finger is moved individually at this joint.

Order of movements

1. Circumduction.
2. Flexion.
3. Extension.
4. Abduction.
5. Adduction.
6. Circumduction.

Interphalangeal joints of fingers and thumb: These are all treated individually with special emphasis being placed on traction separating the joint surfaces. Each joint is firmly held by the beauty therapist above and below its surface localizing the movement and restricting superfluous movement in the other joints.

Order of movements

1. Flexion.
2. Extension.

Saddle joint of thumb: The technique is the same as for the fingers with the palm supinated.

Order of movements

1. Circumduction.
2. Flexion.
3. Extension.
4. Abduction.
5. Adduction.
6. Opposition.
7. Circumduction.

RIGHT LEG

The position of the client remains the same as for the arm movements with the therapist in walk standing and swivelling into stride standing when required.

Hip joint: The full weight of the heavy lower limb is taken by the therapist, placing her left hand underneath the client's knee from the lateral side. The right hand is placed under the heel and sole of the client's right foot. This restricts movements in the ankle joint. The left hand of the therapist must be free to pivot around the knee as the hip is moved the knee is semi-flexed.

Order of movements

1. Circumduction for mobility with the knee in semi-flexion.
2. Flexion.
3. Extension.

4. Abduction; the therapist changes to stride standing with the client's hip and knee flexed.
5. Adduction given in the same position as for abduction.
6. Inward rotation with the leg straight is given by rolling the leg inwards on the couch.
7. Outward rotation by rolling the leg outwards.
8. Circumduction the knee is moved into flexion and the hip joint circled round.

Knee joint: The client and therapist are in the same basic position as for the hip joint movements. The grasp is the same for movements of the knee. The hip is flexed slightly as the knee joint is moved.

Order of movements

1. Flexion.
2. Extension.
3. Medial rotation with the knee in semi-flexion.
4. Lateral rotation with the knee in semi-flexion.

Ankle joint: The grasp is modified and the therapist holds the ankle above the joint with her left hand, placing her right hand along the whole of the sole of the foot, gripping it firmly.

Order of movements

1. Circumduction.
2. Dorsiflexion.
3. Plantarflexion.
4. Inversion.
5. Eversion.
6. Circumduction.

Metatarso-phalangeal and interphalangeal joints of the foot are manipulated in the same way as for the hand. The left hand grasps round the ball of the big toe and the right hand across the back of the toes. Movements of the toes are more restricted than in the hand and care must be taken not to cramp the toes whilst performing the manipulations.

Order of movements

1. Circumduction restricted to the metacarpo-phalangeal joints.
2. Flexion.
3. Extension.
4. Abduction only to metacarpo-phalangeal joints.
5. Adduction only to metacarpo-phalangeal joints.
6. Circumduction to the metacarpo-phalangeal joints.

MOVEMENTS AND GRIPS IN PRONE LYING

Before starting treatment, check the warmth and comfort of the client. Do not use pillows and blankets in this position as they restrict and hamper movements.

HIP JOINT

The therapist stands in stride standing at the side of the thigh on the right of the client. Her right hand and forearm is placed across the sacro-iliac joint and gluteal mass. The left hand and forearm are hooked underneath the front of the right knee and thigh, supporting the weight of the knee, leg, and thigh along the upper arm and forearm. Pressure is applied with the right hand whilst the left hand and arm lifts the leg and thigh backwards into extension.

LUMBAR SPINE

The left hand retains the same firm grasp of the thigh with the leg resting against the upper arm. The right hand of the therapist localizes the movements to the lumbar spine by placing it firmly with pressure over the lower thoracic vertebrae, leaving the lumbar joints free. The client's leg and hip are lifted backwards and the movement is now extended into the lumbar vertebrae.

THORACIC SPINE

The therapist remains in walk standing and moves to the level of the middle of the back. She hooks her right hand and forearm from the back under the client's right axilla, and stretches it across the chest, with the hand holding firmly in the left axilla. Care must be taken not to place the arm across the throat. The left hand localizes each thoracic vertebra with firm pressure, starting from the first working down to the twelfth, whilst the head, shoulders, and back are lifted into extension by the therapist with her right arm. This procedure is then repeated on the other side with hand grips reversed.

SHOULDER GIRDLE

The beauty therapist is in walk standing at the level of the scapulae on the right of the client. Both her arms, the right to the client's right and the left to the client's left, are hooked from the back of the shoulder joint through the client's axillae, to the front of the shoulder joint. They are then brought round gently to the back of the client's neck. Both the client's arms are extended by the therapist, lifting the shoulder joints backwards and pulling the scapulae together. The pectoral muscles across the anterior aspect of the shoulder joints and chest are gently stretched. Care must be taken not to exert a downward thrust with the hands on the back of the neck.

HEAD AND NECK IN LYING

The client is in lying without any support from pillows but she must be warm and comfortable to ensure maximum relaxation. Her shoulders rest across the top of the couch so that the head and neck are entirely free. Ideally, a second therapist should hold the client's shoulders firmly down to provide traction for the moving joints. If this is not possible the weight of the body will provide sufficient anchorage. The beauty therapist takes the stride standing position at the top of the couch behind the client's head. She supports the client's head with one hand; the index finger and thumb are widely apart and are placed round the base of the occiput. Care is taken to ensure that the hair is as much out of the way as possible, otherwise her hand can glide over it, out of the firm grip. The other hand cups the chin carefully. Traction towards the therapist is applied firmly. In order to make the client feel completely confident and secure the grasp must remain consistently firm, taking the full weight of the head throughout the whole treatment. All movements to the head and neck must be slow, rhythmic, and very carefully and gently applied.

Order of movements

1. Circumduction.
2. Flexion.
3. Extension.
4. Right and left side flexion.
5. Rotation to the right with right hand under chin.
6. Rotation to the left with left hand under chin.
7. Circumduction.

Rest is advisable for the client after passive movements to the spine, head, and neck for at least ten minutes on completion of treatment. This will avoid a tendency to light-headedness which the client might feel. She should then be allowed to sit up slowly and dress herself leisurely.

The rate of movements given to the spine, head, and neck should always be moderate, bordering on slow.

Repetition of each movement is unlimited but an average of four to six for each movement is usually given when passive movements are used as a complete treatment in their own right. As little as two repeats of each movement are given if they are included as part of another treatment.

IO. *Active Exercises*

Active exercises are those in which the voluntary muscles are made to contract, and the client performs the movement herself. These movements can be performed freely by the client, or with assistance or resistance provided by gravity, by the therapist, or by equipment.

Exercises are a necessity but they need regular practice to be fully effective in maintaining and improving natural health and beauty. It is never too late to start exercising and never too early to begin. It is important for the beauty therapist to have a basic knowledge about them, and to know exactly what she is trying to achieve and how to do it.

Effects and Uses on the Systems of the Body

MUSCLES

When a muscle contracts it becomes thick and hard, and with repeated exercise the muscle fibres increase in size. The blood supply is increased to the working muscle, feeding and nourishing it, and leaving behind a surplus of food which is stored as muscle bulk (protoplasm). Waste products such as lactic acid are increased and these have a direct action on the walls of the blood vessels in the muscle, dilating them and producing an increased volume of blood to that area. This is called *repletion*. It is said that there is ten times as much blood in a working muscle as in a resting one. Because the working muscles are repleted, blood is taken away from other parts of the body. This is called *depletion* and this factor can be made use of to deplete the blood in the cranium by exercising the trunk and limbs, in the relief of tension headaches. Resting after a meal is to allow the blood to flow fully to the digestive organs. Tone and strength are only built up by muscle activity, and this in turn improves the elasticity and extensibility of the muscles. It is important to bear in mind that muscles both weak and strong if overworked can be strained, fatigued, and weakened. Excess carbon dioxide causes the respiratory centres in the brain to be stimulated in an effort to increase the intake of oxygen. The body temperature is raised and the muscles themselves become warm as the exercises continue, remaining so for quite a while after the activity stops.

BONES

There is an increased blood supply to the bones and joints on active exercise, so that they are nourished and fed. The shape of the bones can be influenced by the pull of muscles so that general exercises ensure proper development. Many daily activities are assymetrical or restricting, and appropriate exercising counterbalances the postural deformities which can occur as a result of limited movement. Whilst muscles are being worked the mobility of the joints is maintained and increased.

CIRCULATION

The venous and lymphatic circulation is improved. As these vessels run over the joints there is a pumping action on them, causing them to be alternately stretched and shortened. This pushes the blood along towards the heart, regurgitation or back flow being prevented by the presence of valves in the veins. The muscles themselves on contraction are squeezed against the veins pressing out the blood and on relaxation allow them to refill. This also aids the venous return to the heart. Sometimes veins are attached to fascia which can compress them. By muscle contraction the fascia is tightened and pressure is relieved, allowing a better blood flow through the part of the vein. The arterial circulation is affected and the flow of blood to different parts of the body is greatly influenced by the active muscles. Blood pressure in the heart is raised and a greater volume of blood is pumped through it, causing it to beat at a faster and stronger rate.

RESPIRATION

The rate and depth of respiration is increased due to the creation of an oxygen need. In this way, the excess carbon dioxide is expelled. Deeper inspiration and expiration increases the mobility of the thorax, strengthening and developing the muscles of respiration at the same time. Whilst the increased circulation promotes the gaseous interchange, the lungs are used and aired to full capacity. Nourishment is brought to the lung tissue by the increased circulation, so increasing their resistance to infection and disease.

DIGESTION, EXCRETION, AND SECRETION

Peristalsis is stimulated due to the action of the abdominal muscles against the involuntary muscle tissue of the digestive tract, and also because of the pressure exerted on the viscera during various movements. This in turn helps the passage of the contents along the alimentary tract whilst the improved tone of the abdominal muscles improves their excretory action. Improved circulation to the abdominal organs promotes secretion of the gastric juices and this again in turn aids digestion and absorption so that all the tissues of the body benefit. More waste products due to increased metabolism are excreted, via the kidneys. As the result of exercise there is an increased production of sweat which helps to rid the body of impurities and excess fluid, cooling the body down as it evaporates on the surface of the skin. The sebaceous glands are stimulated and more sebum being secreted lubricates the skin, providing the body surface with protection from its slight antiseptic properties.

NERVES

Co-ordination, concentration, and co-operation are developed during active exercises. This requires the complicated use of the brain and nervous system, which in order to function efficiently and accurately needs the nourishment that the increased flow of blood brings. Active exercises can be used in such a way to diminish nerve impulses, decreasing all sensations and activities of the body and allowing them to be recharged with energy through rest.

Effects and Uses on Health and Beauty

A marvellous sense of well-being and invigoration comes with exercising and keeping physically fit. Vitality improves, and the woman who seeks a new beauty image will only achieve her objective if she feels one hundred per cent fit. Regular practice of simple movements can help the determined woman to overcome many trivial complaints such as tiredness, tension, stiffness, and even boredom by recharging the systems of the body. Body metabolism is raised by regular exercise and, combined with an appropriate diet, weight can be lost or gained according to the requirements of the client. Exercises can help to keep and improve the lines and contours of the body by fining, trimming, and firming flabby areas, or increasing bulk, filling out the shape where necessary. As the body grows older, muscles tend to contract and shorten. Exercises keep the muscles stretched, supple, and strong. Although the clock cannot be turned back, some of the looks, a lot of the energy, desires, and drives of youth can be regained, keeping the body young and maintaining its activity. Normal functioning of the body is maintained and improved with exercises. In this category comes running for a bus easily, walking upstairs without puffing and blowing, bending and stretching without a backache, full mobility of joints especially for the housewife at spring cleaning time, and ending a busy day for young and old without a screaming headache. As well as toning up the muscles of the body, exercises can help to decrease tension and promote deeper sleep through the art of relaxation, and even help to cure the insomniac. If the client can relax her body, she will be able to relax her mind, and this relaxation of mental tension can take years off the face and off the body, obviating the need to disguise lines and wrinkles under layers of cosmetics. By exercising the body regularly the heart muscle is kept functionally fit, and also ready to cope with any sudden muscular effort, or emergency. It is important to prevent the heart from becoming weak and sluggish; like a faithful dog it needs exercising regularly every day to cope efficiently in a time of stress. If the client is in poor muscular tone then in those muscles exercised, she may experience up to several days afterwards, a certain amount of muscle ache, tenderness, and stiffness. This wears off gradually and decreases as the muscles are strengthened, toned, and used through their full range of movement, with carefully planned exercises. After half an hour of either localized or general exercises the client should feel glowing, radiant, pleasantly tired, but refreshed with eyes shining and bright. A steam bath or sauna followed by a massage and rest completes, together with the exercises, one of the most revitalizing overall beauty treatments available. Popular with both men and women, young and old alike, regardless of shape or size, these basic ingredients for health and beauty have remained virtually the same for centuries.

CONTRA-INDICATIONS

1. When medically ill-advised.
2. High blood pressure or any acute heart condition.
3. Arterio-sclerosis (hardening of the arteries); usually the client is elderly and should be aware of the condition.
4. High temperatures.
5. Extreme cases of debility, general tiredness, and weakness.
6. Any advanced disease in the body.
7. Recent injuries.
8. Acute inflammatory conditions of joints, such as rheumatoid arthritis where the joints, particularly the smaller ones, would be hot, swollen, and very painful to move.

9. Fevers.
10. Health reasons, unless medically recommended.

Some Mechanics of Body Movement

LEVERS

In the body the bones are used as levers to lift the limbs or different parts quickly, easily, and in a well balanced manner. The joints act as the fulcrum, the point about which the lever moves, and the power or force required to lift the weight of the limbs is provided by the muscles. Depending upon what action or movement is required, the balance, power, and speed can be altered by the position of the levers in relation to the fulcrum and the power.

There are three classes of levers:

CLASS OF LEVERS

The classes of levers are illustrated in Figure 18 as follows:

1. The fulcrum or joint lies somewhere between the weight to be moved and the power. For example, in plantar flexion of the foot, the fulcrum is the ankle joint; the weight is the foot and the power is the insertion of tendo-Achilles. The longer the distance from the fulcrum to the power, the easier the movement. The movement is more difficult when the distance from the weight to the fulcrum is increased.
2. The weight lies between the power and the fulcrum. For example, in standing on tiptoes, the fulcrum is the metatarso-phalangeal joints, the power from the calf muscles inserted into the calcaneum, and the weight is that of the body which falls on to the tarsals. Little effort is required in these movements.
3. The power lies between the fulcrum and the weight. For example, in knee extension, the fulcrum is the knee joint, the power is the insertion of the quadriceps muscles into the tibial tubercle lifting the weight of the leg and foot. Much effort is required in these movements. Almost every movement in the body falls into this class.

B.M.—7*

The distance from the fulcrum to the point where the power is applied is called the weight lever, and by lengthening the weight lever in free movements the movement can be made more difficult; also by increasing the resistance with added weight and placing them further away from the moving joint.

FIGURE 18.   Levers

AXES AND PLANES OF MOVEMENTS

Movements of the body take place round an imaginary line called the axis. The axis is in the joint. Some joints are capable of producing several movements round different axes. These movements take place on an imaginary flat surface called a plane. There are three axes and three planes of movement.

AXES

1. *Frontal* or transverse axis is round a line from side to side of the body which lies parallel with the forehead or the coronary suture in the skull.
2. *Saggital* axis is a line from front to back of the body parallel with the saggital suture in the skull.
3. *Vertical* or longitudinal axis is a line drawn through the body from the head to the feet.

PLANES

1. *Frontal* plane is a flat surface parallel with the face and coronary suture.
2. *Saggital* plane is a surface parallel with the saggital suture.
3. *Horizontal* plane is one which is parallel to the dorsum of the foot and the ground.

EXAMPLES

1. Trunk side flexion (bending the body sideways from the waist) takes place round the saggital axis on a frontal plane.
2. Trunk rotation (twisting the body round from the waist) takes place round a vertical axis on a horizontal plane.
3. Trunk flexion (bending the body forwards from the waist) takes place round the frontal axis on a saggital plane.

GRAVITY

The force of gravity is the force or pull which the earth exerts on objects towards its own centre. The force acts at right angles to the earth's surface, so that if an object is dropped from a height it will fall perpendicularly downwards.

CENTRE OF GRAVITY OF THE BODY

The point on which the pull of gravity is the strongest in the human body is its centre of gravity. If the human body could be held straight like a plank of wood, it would be the point at which the plank balances over a pivot. In the body this point normally falls in front of the second or third sacral vertebra, but depends upon the shape, size, and weight of the individual. Each part of the body has its own centre of gravity.

LINE OF GRAVITY

The direction in which gravity pulls the body is called the line of gravity. This imaginary line, either side of which the weight must be equal, normally falls from the centre of the vortex of the skull to a point midway between the feet.

From the anatomical position, this line falls from the skull in front of the ears, through the cervical and thoracic vertebrae, through the bodies of the lumbar vertebrae, hip joint, just behind the knee joint, and just in front of the ankle joint, to the point between the feet. Any movement from the normal postural attitude alters its position.

By altering the centre and line of gravity of the body exercises can be made more difficult or easier. Balance, co-ordination, and posture are also affected.

RANGE OF MOVEMENT

Movements are produced by the contraction of muscles. The extent of the movement produced is called the range or path of movement of the muscles. There are four ranges of movement:

1. *Full range* is from the most stretched point of a muscle to its most contracted point.
2. *Inner range* is from its midpoint of contraction to its most contracted point.
3. *Outer range* is from the most stretched point to the midpoint of contraction.
4. *Middle range* is from the almost fully stretched point to the almost fully contracted point.

USES OF THE RANGES

General strengthening exercises are given through full range. Toning, shortening, and strengthening exercises are given in inner range.

For lengthening and maintaining strength, outer range exercises are used.

Everyday functional movements are usually performed in middle range and there is a danger of stiffness in the joints and muscles if their full range of movement is not maintained properly.

MUSCLE WORK

Muscles work in three different ways when they contract. They normally work against the resistance of an outside force such as gravity. Weights and apparatus can be used if available.

1. *Concentric* muscle work is that in which the muscle becomes shorter and thicker; the origin and insertion move nearer together. Concentric muscle work produces heat in the muscles and body. It is the hardest, though most common, form of all resisted exercises. It can be used in all ranges of movement.

2. *Eccentric* muscle work is that in which the muscle lengthens and hardens, the origin and insertion being drawn further away from each other, paying out against a resistance (gravity). Eccentric muscle work is considered to be easier than concentric muscle work. It produces less heat in the body but more work, which has the tendency to make the client hold her breath and feel tired. It can be used in all ranges.

3. *Static* muscle work is that in which the muscle contracts and becomes hard and thick, with neither lengthening nor shortening and no movement. Little heat or muscle work is produced by static muscle contractions. They are given to hold positions, particularly in the correction of poor posture, where with repeated holdings of the corrected position, the postural sense is educated in the client, forming new improved automatic habits. Static contractions for a short period of time are the easiest form of muscle work; over a long period of time they produce fatigue. They are used as a starter to strengthen very weak muscles, and to strengthen endurance for functional activities.

Some Important Points for Exercise Schemes

1. The age, condition, occupation, and sex of the client are the first considerations.

2. If the scheme of exercises is a general one then exercises for all parts of the body should be included. Easier exercises begin and end the treatment, with harder ones in the middle.

3. Exercises which use the same muscles or muscle groups should not be given consecutively. In this way overwork of any one muscle is avoided.

4. It is important to vary the exercises in each treatment to avoid boredom. Interest must be stimulated and maintained. Music can be a helpful means to help rhythm and grace of movement. A modulated voice, with the exercise command well executed, can be most effective. Balance and co-ordination exercises always add interest and liven up the treatment. If more than one client is treated at once, some form of competitive exercises or games should be included.

5. Special exercises for specific problems should be emphasized if included in a general scheme of exercises.

6. A goal should be aimed for, if possible, to encourage the client to persevere and practise home exercises. These should be taught and repeated at the end of the session. The client must know exactly what exercises to do and how to do them. They should consist of natural functional movements.

7. Depending upon the kind of problem requiring attention, the choice of time should be considered. For example, relaxation exercises could be given late in the day if they are to help insomnia. Active exercises would never be given after a meal.

8. Exercises for health reasons are only given when medical permission is granted.

9. The first sessions should be short and sweet. As the muscles strengthen, the sessions can last longer by including more exercises, and repeating each exercise more often. An accurate chart must be kept, noting all details of the exercises.

10. Mobility exercises are a vital starter for all schemes; these help to warm up the muscles and loosen the joints. Muscles and joints which are cold and stiff can be torn and easily strained if they are not warmed up first. Five to ten minutes would be devoted to warming up.

11. Breathing and postural correction should begin and end all schemes of exercises. They can and should be interspersed freely throughout the whole session. The breathing exercises will give the client a chance to rest and recoup a little energy. Sometimes the exercises can be combined with breathing instruction.

12. At the end of the session the client should feel pleasantly tired but not exhausted, and facilities should be available for her to be able to relax lying down for at least fifteen minutes if required. The client should be suitably dressed in unrestricting clothes; the room should be airy, warm, and bright.

Order of a General Scheme of Exercises

A basic general scheme of exercises should include all the principal muscle groups of the body. Not more than twelve to sixteen movements are advised. If the scheme is designed for a strenuous keep fit class, then the mobility exercises alone at the beginning of the session could last for up to twenty minutes. The following skeleton table for a simple scheme of exercises will be found a useful guide to follow, bearing in mind the above points.

SKELETON TABLES OF EXERCISES

1. Breathing exercise.
2. Postural correction exercise.
3. Arm mobility exercise.
4. Leg mobility exercise.
5. Head and neck mobility exercise.
6. Trunk mobility exercise.
7. Straight abdominal exercise.
8. Back exercise.
9. Oblique abdominal exercise.

10. Back exercise.
11. Arm exercise.
12. Leg exercise.
13. Breathing exercise.
14. Postural correction exercise.

PROGRESSION OF EXERCISES

The means by which exercises are made more difficult is the progression of exercises. There are many ways in which to achieve this purpose.

1. *Starting* positions can be altered. The basic starting positions are lying, kneeling, sitting, standing, and hanging. There are many variations derived from these positions. By making the base of the starting position smaller the exercise becomes harder. By complicating the basic starting position, bringing into play a larger number of joints and muscles, the difficulty of the exercise is increased. For instance, lying is the easiest position as it has the largest base. Little effort, if any, is required from the muscles and joints to maintain it. Crook lying, or lying with the knees bent, is a progression, for the size of the base has diminished and also some effort is required to keep the knees bent. It is easier to do an exercise in stride standing (feet apart) than it is in close standing (feet together), or toe standing where the size of the base has now been considerably reduced and many more muscles are brought into action.

2. *Repetition* of movements is helpful, also holding the action statically for longer periods whilst performing another exercise if required.

3. *Altering* the centre of gravity by raising it makes the exercise harder. For example, trunk bending forwards is made more difficult with the arms stretched above the head.

4. *Lengthening* the lever increases the weight and resistance to the movement. For example, raising the arms sideways to shoulder level is easier with the fingertips on the shoulders and the elbows bent than with the arms fully stretched sideways.

5. *Removing* the stability of the more fixed point (origin) of the working muscle is difficult. For example, double leg lifting in the lying position becomes more difficult if the hands are not holding on to a support.

6. *Increasing* the resistance to a muscle to its maximum is helpful. The resistance can be provided by apparatus, including springs, weights, pulleys, or by the therapist's manual resistance or by self resistance.

7. *Asymmetrical* exercises can be added whereby the limbs perform different actions at the same time. These can progress by combining asymmetrical movements of the trunk, head, arms, and legs into one exercise.

8. *Co-ordination* exercises can increase the difficulty and perfect the movements. These can be done by combining a series of actions of the trunk, head, arms, and legs into one exercise. The client has to concentrate throughout on performing the complicated exercise and maintaining a good starting position.

9. *Balance* exercises performed slowly are extremely difficult. They also improve co-ordination and posture at the same time, and are invaluable in any scheme of exercises designed to improve the general appearance.

STARTING POSITIONS

It is important to consider in what position the exercises are going to be performed. In massage the aim is to make the client as comfortable as possible before commencing treatment. With exercises the aim is to ensure that the best possible effect is produced from the exercise, according to the requirements and capabilities of the client, bearing in mind that the details of correct posture are of vital importance throughout. There are five fundamental positions used in remedial exercises, the principles of which can be used for cosmetic exercises. They are lying, sitting, standing, kneeling, hanging. From these positions, other positions are modified, and these are known as the derived positions. The starting positions should be carefully considered when treating clients, and checked and corrected throughout the whole treatment. If this is not done, then the posture of the client may remain poor, and whilst the movements are being performed, muscles other than those used in holding the starting positions will be brought into play, defeating the aim.

LYING POSITION

A wide flat surface should be used. The client lies on her back with the arms resting by her sides. The legs should be relaxed, falling into slight outward rotation with the feet in relaxed plantar flexion. Her head will be back with chin tucked in, chest slightly out, and shoulders gently back.

SITTING POSITION

A stool or chair of suitable height is used. The thighs are supported from the ischial tuberosities to the back of the knees. The legs must be at a right angle to the thighs with the feet flat and slightly apart pointing forwards. The trunk is held upright, head up, chin in, shoulders back but relaxed, arms held at the sides with wrist and fingers gently extended.

STANDING POSITION

The client stands with heels together and toes very slightly apart. Head, shoulders, and arms are held as in the sitting position. The abdominal muscles are pulled in, the seat muscles tightened, and the knees straight.

KNEELING POSITION

Kneeling on the floor, with the knees placed slightly apart, the feet are plantar flexed and the toes bent under. The thighs and trunk should be directly over the knees; the rest of the position the same as for standing.

HANGING POSITION

Taken on wall bars, or a horizontal bar, the client's feet must be just off the floor. The hands are pronated, gripping the bar, and the arms at least shoulder-width apart with the body hanging in a straight line. The feet should be in plantar flexion.

Muscle Work, Effects, and Uses of the Fundamental Positions

LYING

Lying is the easiest starting position. The base is large and no muscle work is necessary to maintain the position. It can, however, restrict breathing slightly, and would be contra-indicated for clients who need to see the movements of the limbs whilst performing them. It is a good position in which to teach relaxation, to exercise weak muscles, and to exercise after massage when this position is already used. When age and ability are a consideration, this position is also used. Lying is not a good position for anyone with a lordosis (hollow back).

SITTING

Sitting fixes the legs, hips, and pelvis, localizing movements to the upper part of the body making it easier for them to move. It is a safe steady position because the centre of gravity is low and the base is firm and large. It is a convenient starting position because it can be readily adapted to suit any requirements in a limited space. Clients who are unable to balance very well, perhaps elderly clients, can be given a variety of exercises to all parts of the body, head, and limbs which can progress into standing. Some clients unable to stand for long periods will find this an excellent position to work in, and will be encouraged to practise exercises at home if this position is adopted. Resistances can be added to movements in this position.

Muscles involved in maintaining this position are the flexors and extensors of the neck, the long back muscles, the adductors of the scapulae, the abdominal muscles and hip flexors, the extensors of the hips and knees, and the plantar flexors of the feet.

STANDING

Standing is the hardest of all the fundamental positions to maintain. It is a good position in which to start with warming-up exercises as there is no restriction of movement, all joints and muscles being free. The client will be alerted and awakened in this position. Concentration and co-ordination is necessary to maintain the position because the centre of gravity is high and the base is small. The majority of clients, except the elderly, should be able to cope with any exercise given in the fundamental standing position.

Muscles involved are the same as for the sitting position in the head and trunk, the hip and knee extensors more so, the adductors of the legs and the muscles in the soles of the feet (the interossei and lumbricals), and an interplay between the plantar and dorsi flexors. The muscle work in standing relies upon the balance of the bones on each other, and upon the postural balance between the muscles on the front and back of the body.

KNEELING

Kneeling is a steadier position than standing but not a particularly comfortable one because of the pressure on the knees. It is not suitable for clients who have a lordosis, but good trunk movements and free head and arm movements can be used in this position. Although the base is large and the centre of gravity low, this position is not often used.

Muscle work involved is the same as for standing, except that the hip extensors must work more strongly to counterbalance the tendency to fall forwards. The intrinsic muscles of the feet do not work and the knee flexors work harder to maintain the balance.

HANGING

Hanging is a position used for particularly strong clients and where strengthening exercises are required to be given to the limbs and trunk. The spine and ligaments are stretched and, where postural problems need attention, hanging is an excellent starting position to stretch out mild deformities. It is particularly useful for young clients who should be able to perform strong work, and also where postural conditions are not combined with respiratory complications. The normally healthy client would feel quite invigorated after exercises given in hanging.

Muscles required to work maintaining the hanging position are the flexors of the fingers, the wrist flexors and extensors, the flexors of the elbow, the adductors of the shoulder and scapulae (latissimus dorsi, pectoralis major, rhomboids, and the middle fibres of trapezius).

N.B. This position is contra-indicated for all older clients or whenever there is any form of weakness, after operations, and in any form of lung disease. Care must be taken, in all the positions during and after exercises, that the client does not become dizzy. Stretching on the spine can cause a sensation of dizziness, particularly in hanging.

DERIVED POSITIONS

Basically derived positions are modifications of the fundamental positions by changing the positions of the arms, legs, head, and trunk. There are many derived positions in which exercises are performed. Here are some derived positions described in detail for use later in the chapter. The advantage of using the descriptive terminology is to cut out unnecessary repetitive and lengthy description. In a way it can be likened to shorthand. Exercises and movements today are generally based on the more natural positions of the body.

STANDING

Stride standing: The feet are placed two foot lengths apart, the weight being evenly distributed between each foot. A steady firm position.

Walk standing: One foot is placed in front of the other, two foot lengths between the heels. Weight must be evenly distributed. Used very much together with stride standing in massage.

Curtsy standing: The hip and knee joints are flexed to right angles, with trunk kept upright; knees are apart.

LYING

Prone lying: Client lies face down fully supported, or with head to one side.

Crook lying: Client lies with both knees bent, feet flat on the floor.

SITTING

Long sitting: Client sits on floor with legs stretched out and knees together. Back must be erect.

Crook sitting: Client sits on the floor with the knees bent according to comfort and requirements. Important to check upright position of head and back.

KNEELING

Prone kneeling: The body is parallel to the floor and is supported by the hands which are placed shoulder-width apart and vertical, hands pointing forwards, the knees are flexed at right angles, hip-width.

Programme of Exercises

There is little need to point out again the value of exercising. Most women welcome and grasp the chance to improve the contours of their body. Gone are the days when big bosoms, generous hips, and spreading thighs represented Man's pinnacle of beauty. Now it seems that it is desirable to have a firm bustline, trim waistline, flat tummy, slim arms, and slender tapering legs. By the means of exercise much can be done to achieve this ideal image. There need be no fear of turning into a muscular unfeminine figure; one has only to look at the female athletes of ice skating, tennis, or gymnastics to see that even after a lifetime devoted to sport the fair sex remains frankly feminine.

Like anything that is worth doing exercises require perseverance, practice, and patience. It is no good teaching the client some marvellous exercises if she is only going to do them once or twice a week with the beauty therapist. She must become sufficiently inspired and interested enough by the therapist to practise them at home.

Ideally they should be practised at least three times a day for a minimum of ten minutes at any one time. The client could be instructed to rise ten minutes earlier in the morning and retire ten minutes earlier at night, for the sole purpose of practising the exercises. Midday or when convenient would be a good time for the third ten minutes set aside to practise home exercises. Not more than four exercises should be given, otherwise there is a tendency to forget the detailed instruction of each exercise. Two or three minutes spent carefully and thoroughly on each exercise is not much to ask the client to do.

Simple home exercises that can be incorporated into a daily routine anywhere and at any time are another means of achieving the client's co-operation in helping herself with her beauty project, if she is not too keen on the ten-minutes-a-time routine. For example, instead of climbing upstairs one at a time, increase this to two at a time, to improve all leg muscles. For the waistline, suggest to the client that every time she passes through a doorway, she stands still and touches her toes twenty times before moving on. If there are too many doors, select only certain doors and apply it to those. Whenever the client washes her hands or works at the sink, instruct her to push hard together the palms of the hands ten times to exercise the chest muscles, firming the bustline and upper arm. Whilst sitting chatting on the telephone, lift the body just off the chair as though standing up, and then sit down again; no help with the hands. This last exercise is a bit disconcerting as concentration in listening to the person at the other end of the line tends to wane in the effort to perform the exercise, but what price is that to pay for a new hip- and thigh-line! Most important of all is the posture, which the client should be made aware of whenever she sees her reflection in a mirror or a shop window. An erect posture improves all contours automatically; the client must remember that all she has to do for a good posture regained quickly is merely to lift up her head with the chin in, pull back the shoulders, and pull in the tummy. Many chores require periods of standing, either at home, at work, or even waiting for a bus. Here is a good exercise for the client to practise whilst standing, to exercise the internal muscles of the pelvis.

Cross one leg over the other and squeeze the seat muscles and tops of the legs tightly together as though trying not to spend a penny. Relax and change over legs. Very simply done without fuss, this exercise will help to prevent low backache and dragging pains in this area. The more it is performed the merrier, but up to about ten contractions each side at a time would be ideal.

MUSCLE BUILDING

Muscles can be built up considerably by exercise. If bulk is required for any one particular area, then usually weight lifting, or exercising the specific muscle against some form of resistance is necessary. The therapist must measure the girth of that particular muscle or area before treatment, and then regularly once a week. A careful and accurate weight lifting chart must be made, recording details of weights lifted or resistances used. Concentric muscle work through full range is used. A general guide would be, for normally healthy muscles, to start off with a minimum weight, lifting it five times, contracting the required muscle. The static holdings in between each contraction must not be neglected. The muscle is then rested before this procedure is repeated twice more making a total of fifteen contractions. If the muscle shows any sign of fatigue, such as trembling or an inability to contract fully or sustain the contraction statically, then the programme must be revised. Cut the basic number of contractions down to three and build up from there. The maximum number of contractions should reach ten, making a final total of thirty contractions at any one time. The weight depends on the strength of the muscle, but a one-pound or two-pound (half or one kilogramme) weight to begin with should be easy to lift for the normal healthy muscle. If proper weight-lifting equipment is not available, improvisations can easily be made by self-resisting exercises, or with the therapist resisting, or with books, or tins of food, that could be brought and previously weighed by the therapist from home. These should be firmly attached to the right point on the lever of the body required to be lifted by the specific muscle or muscle group in question. Weight lifting for muscle building needs to be precisely followed. When the first weight is easily lifted ten times, then, and only then, can the weight be increased. The number of contractions is decreased to five again, and the procedure repeated and continued accordingly till the required effect has been produced. Self-resisting and therapist-resisting exercises are not an accurate means of weight lifting for muscle building. They are better than nothing, but are mainly used in free exercises when a little extra resistance other than gravity is required. The repetition of exercises will strengthen tone and will firm up the muscles to some extent, but, for a marked increase in bulk and girth, some form of regular progressive resistance must be added to the contracting muscle. These exercises should be practised daily at least once, and twice if possible, to see speedier results. At the end of six weeks there should be a marked improvement in the size of the muscle. Three months' diligent practising will produce excellent results for all schemes of exercising.

Explanation, Command, and Cycle of Exercise

Before the client is asked to perform the exercise, or exercises, the therapist must give a clear and precise explanation of what is required. If necessary, she should passively move the client in an attempt to show her, or should demonstrate the exercise herself first. The client is told what starting position to adopt, then the exercise explanation is given. This deals with correction of the starting position, which part of the body is to be moved, what movement is required, where to move it, and, by a clear command, when to move it. The cycle of the exercise continues because the contraction must be sustained in strengthening exercises by a static contraction for stamina, then must be returned to the starting position, and finally relaxed. For example, if the client is required to exercise the abdominal muscles in back lying with both knees bent onto the chest, then stretched in the air, lowered six inches (15 cm), lifted again, then legs bent, and down into the back lying starting position, after explaining this, the following commands would be given: 'Lie on your back (legs straight); both knees on to your chest, bend; both legs into the air, lift; both legs six inches lower, hold; both legs upwards, lift; both knees slowly, bend; both legs downwards, stretch; and relax.' This is quite a complicated exercise which must be clearly explained. Less involved exercises must be just as precisely delivered to the client when teaching her the exercises. Once she has understood what it is she is required to do, detailed explanations of exercises become superfluous and the abbreviated commands only are used. For example, a simple arm exercise in stride standing would be taught as follows: 'Stand with feet apart (head up, chin in, shoulders back); both arms forwards to shoulder level, lift; hold; lower; relax!'

STRENGTHENING EXERCISE

When giving strengthening exercises, part of the cycle of the exercise is to order the holding of the contraction before giving the order to return the limb to the original position and to relax. At this point a reminder to breathe (not to hold the breath) is very often necessary. This is where the benefit of interspersing breathing exercises proves to be not only valuable in itself, but a useful resting point. The length of time that the contraction is held is entirely up to the judgment of the therapist and the condition of the client's muscles. Generally speaking, a good guide would be to start off holding a contraction to the slow count of three (roughly three seconds). This can be increased by one second gradually, as the muscles strengthen. Different muscles will be able to sustain their contractions for longer periods of time than others, depending on their strength. To start with, the exercise itself should be repeated about six times.

Gradually the repetition is increased as the muscles gain in strength to a maximum of ten contractions. These guides apply to the normal average client. Obviously someone who is particularly weak, or excessively fit, would need special considerations. Relaxations of the muscles and the body after each contraction is an integral part of exercising, but it is important to understand that, until the limb or part of the body moved has been returned to the starting position, the command to relax is not given, otherwise it could be taken literally. For example, if a leg was still held up in the air and the command to relax given, the client might just let it flop down, causing bruising and strain. Apart from that fact, returning the limb to the original position belongs to the cycle of the exercise. Very often it involves using the muscles eccentrically on the return journey, and as such must not be overlooked. An experienced therapist should be able to balance and work out exactly how and in which range the muscles are required to be used, in order to achieve the maximum result.

MOBILITY EXERCISES

Mobility exercises should be performed quickly, loosely, and freely without static holdings. The same movement should be repeated several times consecutively before the order to rest is given. A breathing exercise is more essential here before continuing with the same exercise several times again. Three or four repetitions of the same mobility exercise cycle is ample before moving on to another one, bearing in mind that the main function of mobility exercises is to warm up and loosen the body or parts through as full a range as possible prior to giving strengthening exercises.

Mobility exercises can be readily changed into strengthening exercises by reducing the speed of movement and adding a static holding of the contraction as explained previously. The variations possible on any one particular exercise, for any one muscle, are enormous by using different starting positions, ranges of movement, and muscle work. Exercise permutations are quite a fascinating study if not quite as numerous as football perms. The beauty therapist should be able to work out for herself a balanced scheme of progressive and interesting exercises. The exercises have been described as though directed towards the beauty therapist and for her to try out first, generally speaking, throughout the book.

Posture

A good professional model glides along gracefully and erect. Every movement, having been carefully considered, is elegantly made. It is all a question of correct posture remembered and practised until it becomes second nature. A client does not have to be a model to walk tall. Even the plainest client can look most becoming if her posture is impeccable. Some people seem to be born with a natural swing of the hips, straight shoulders, and head held high without giving it a second thought. For the client whose stance leaves much to be desired, a careful examination of the spine is essential. This will reveal exactly what kind of postural correction is indicated during the course of exercises. Perhaps only slight correction is required, or maybe a more rigorous and specific scheme of exercises will have to be devised. Good posture relies upon the interplay and co-ordination of the flexor and extensor groups of muscles in the body. If one group of muscles becomes weak or too strong, then the whole postural balance is thrown out of line. Bad posture can lead to many side effects, including postural defects of the spine, which, apart from destroying good looks, bring their own set of problems to the body. A full-length mirror is extremely useful in teaching the client postural correction. She can see herself corrected, feel the correction, remember the correction, and recheck the new position again in the mirror.

INSPECTION OF THE SPINE FROM THE BACK

Make sure that the client is suitably dressed so that the whole spine is visible. Bra and pants would be adequate. The light must be good and the room warm. The beauty therapist stands behind the client to check the general posture. The client is in standing.

1. The general outline and stance of the client are first noted.
2. The ears should be level and the neck straight.
3. The shoulders should be level.
4. The medial borders of the scapulae should be at an even distance from the spine. The inferior angles of the scapulae should be level and lying flat against the back of the chest wall.
5. The angle at the waist should be evenly curved and not more apparent on one side than the other with neither hip higher than the other.
6. The ribs will be evenly spaced and not closer together on one side nor farther apart on the other.
7. The soft structures on either side should not show any signs of shortening nor abnormal signs of lengthening on the opposite side.
8. The spines themselves should be down the centre of the back, and if a finger is gently rubbed down the spines of the vertebrae they will redden, and the curve of the spine will be seen clearly.
9. The gluteal folds should be even and at the same height.
10. The arms will hang evenly near to the sides of the body.
11. Knock knees, bandy legs, or flat feet are noted.

INSPECTION FROM THE FRONT

1. Head should be high and held back, with chin tucked in and neck straight.
2. Shoulder and ear levels should be even.
3. Shoulders should be slightly back with chest and thorax out and broad.
4. Arms and hands relaxed down by the sides of the thigh, not too far forwards.
5. Even waist-line with iliac crests level.
6. Abdominal muscles slightly retracted.
7. Legs and knees straight, feet facing forwards or slightly apart with heels together.

If all these points are correct, the posture of the client should be excellent. However, what is a good posture for one person can be bad posture for another.

ACTIVE CORRECTION OF POSTURE BY THE THERAPIST

1. See that the client's head is up with chin in.
2. Shoulders back, but down and relaxed.
3. Chest out.
4. Arms should lie in centre of thighs by the sides.
5. Abdominal muscles pulled in.
6. Seat muscles tight and tucked in.
7. Knees straight but not tightly braced back.
8. Inner and outer sides of feet gripping floor with arches of foot raised.

ACTIVE STATIC MUSCLE CONTRACTIONS TO MAINTAIN CORRECT POSTURE

Static holding of a good postural position is important to learn if correction is necessary and if it requires only a simple reminder to put right. Sometimes the client can easily correct a bad posture herself and the following static corrections would be given in the corrected standing position. The therapist would tell the client how to do the following statically.

1. Brace arm and leg muscles, hold, relax.
2. Brace neck and back of shoulder muscles, hold, relax.
3. Brace back muscles, hold, relax.
4. Brace back muscles and abdominal muscles, hold, relax.
5. Brace all muscles, hold, relax.

GENERAL BACK STRENGTHENING EXERCISES FOR IMPROVEMENT OF ERECT POSTURE

Position: Prone lying.

Muscle work: Concentric and static holding of all back muscles in inner range.

1. Lift head and shoulders off the floor (or couch); look down with chin tucked in; hold the position, lower, relax.

2. Lift right straight leg backwards, hold, lower, relax. Repeat with left leg.
3. Place both hands under forehead, in forehead rest prone lying, lift head, hands, arms, and elbows backwards off the floor, hold, lower, relax.
4. Lift both straight legs backwards, hold, lower, relax.
5. Stretch arms above head on the floor, lift right arm and straight left leg backwards off the floor, hold, lower, relax. Repeat with opposite arm and leg.

SPECIFIC POSTURAL CONDITIONS

Any postural condition, other than that which can be corrected actively by simple postural exercises, really needs specialized attention outside the sphere of the beauty therapist. However, in the course of treatment, there will be clients who require a course of exercises and yet have specific spinal defects. It is in these cases that the beauty therapist's guidance will be of great assistance. Therefore, it is essential for the beauty therapist to familiarize herself with conditions that may possibly confront her. She must be able to recognize them whilst examining the spine so that only corrective exercises are given in the course of treatment, and not exercises inadvertently prescribed which would be contra-indicated for the condition. If it is merely a matter of habitual bad posture, then corrective exercises will eventually give the client the right idea of the correct posture. It is as well to bear in mind that no two individuals are alike, and that each body type has its own characteristic postural make-up.

PELVIC TILT

The pelvic tilt is the angle which is made between a horizontal line and a line drawn from the top of the symphysis pubis to the sacral promontory. This angle varies, being greater in the female than in the male. The amount of movement possible in the pelvic angle depends upon the pelvic ligaments and joints. During pregnancy the ligaments are relaxed and movements in all these joints is increased so the pelvic tilt will alter, often increasing considerably. If the pelvis tilts forwards too much, the lumbar vertebrae can become hyperextended; if it tilts backwards too far, the curve in the lumbar vertebrae can flatten.

EXERCISES FOR PELVIC TILT

Position: sitting or standing.

1. Pull in the abdominal muscles tightly, tucking in the seat muscles and tightening them at the same time. Relax the abdominal muscles and push the buttocks backwards, hollowing the bottom of the back. Repeat this several times.

Position: curtsy standing.

1. Place one hand on the tummy, one hand on the sacrum. Pull in the tummy muscles, tucking the seat in. Relax the abdominal muscles and arch the base of the spine forwards, sticking out the seat.

   Really let the client feel the pelvis tilting backwards and forwards in this position.

Position: prone kneeling.

1. Hump the back up at the sacro–lumbar region by pulling in the abdominal muscles, tightening and tucking in the seat muscles. This decreases the angle.
2. Hollow the back at the sacro–lumbar region, letting it curve downwards by pushing up the buttocks into the air. This increases the angle.
3. Hump and hollow alternately, quickly for mobilization of the lumbar spine and slowly for strengthening.

LORDOSIS

In this condition the client will appear to have a hollow back at the lumbar region. There is an exaggerated curve forwards in the lumbar region. Here the pelvic tilt is greatly increased forwards. The abdominal muscles and hamstrings are stretched and lengthened, with the lumbar muscles shortened and gluteal muscles weakened. The aim would be to give corrective exercises which would shorten and strengthen the abdominal and hamstring muscles, also to strengthen the gluteal muscles mobilizing the lumbar spine at the same time.

EXERCISES FOR LORDOSIS

Position: stride standing.

1. Quickly bend the trunk and arms forward and down to touch the toes, taking care not to stretch too far back when raising up again. Repeat this exercise quickly several times for mobility.
2. Quickly for mobility, bend the trunk and arms over and down to the right foot, raise upwards, and repeat to the left.

Position: any position.

1. Abdominal contractions—pulling in the abdominal muscles tucking in the seat, tilting the pelvis backwards.

Position: crook lying, taking care to see that the lumbar spine is flat on the bed or floor.

1. Lift head and shoulders off the bed, slowly curling forwards until sitting up, straightening out the legs at the same time; stretch forwards to touch the toes. Lie down again in reverse order and repeat as for strengthening.

Position: stride standing.

1. Slowly bend over to touch toes; slowly stand up again.

KYPHOSIS

In this condition, the normal backward curve of the spine in the thoracic region is exaggerated. Generally speaking, the client will have a poking chin and rounded shoulders as well. It is very often attributed to habitual bad posture but there are many other causes. The pectoral muscles are tight and shortened with the upper back muscles weak and over-stretched. The aim is to mobilize and loosen the tightened structures and strengthen those which are stretched, and to correct the posture.

EXERCISES FOR KYPHOSIS

Position: sitting.

1. Bend the head and shoulders forwards to touch the knees, and quickly sit up again.
2. Shoulders backwards circling round.
3. Rotation of the trunk. Place fingertips on shoulders, bend forwards twisting over to the right knee, across to the left knee, and up into the sitting position. Repeat this movement round in the opposite direction. This can be used for mobility and strength.
4. With fingertips still on the shoulders, twist the trunk forwards to try and touch the right elbow on to the left knee. Repeat to the opposite side with the left elbow.

Position: hanging (with back on bars or free).

1. Hang on the bars and just lift the feet off the floor by dorsi-flexing the ankles.
2. Arch the body off the bars, by pressing the heels and head backwards, pulling back the shoulders at the same time.

Position: prone lying.

1. All strengthening exercises given earlier for general postural correction, using the longitudinal and transverse back muscles.
2. Head, shoulders, and legs backwards off the floor lifting, taking care to see that the client's chin is tucked in; hold this position, lower, and relax.

Position: sitting and standing.

1. Head extensions, that is, pulling in the chin and pressing and pulling back the head.
2. Head nodding forwards and backwards, correcting chin position.

KYPHO-LORDOSIS

This is a combination of the two latter conditions; one rarely goes without the other.

When exercises for the back are given, the lumbar spine should be corrected first so that the lordosis is not increased. When abdominal exercises are given, the thoracic region and shoulders should be straight and back so that the kyphosis is not encouraged.

EXERCISES FOR KYPHO-LORDOSIS

Position: sitting.
1. Pulling in the tummy muscles and tightening the gluteal muscles of the seat, swing both arms forwards, backwards, and upwards several times.
2. Lift the right knee upwards and at the same time stretch the left arm forwards and upwards above the head. Change position with the opposite arm and leg.

Position: stride standing.
1. Bend forwards to touch floor and walk forwards on the floor five paces with the hands and five paces backwards. Straighten up and correct the posture.
2. Bend forwards to touch floor and walk forwards with hands and feet five paces and five paces backwards.

Position: standing or sitting.
1. Turn the trunk and head round to the right from the waist and stretch the right arm backwards. Change to stretch round to the left following the trunk turning with the left arm.
2. Circling both arms backwards in large circles pulling in the tummy muscles, and stretching the shoulders backwards at the same time.

FLAT BACK

This condition is rarely seen but here the pelvis is tilted backwards, the lumbar spines are flat, and the hamstrings are shortened. The client may appear to be very erect and square-shouldered because the natural curves of the spine are almost ironed out. The aim would be to mobilize the spine and stretch the shortened muscles. Exercises for mobility would include humping and hollowing as explained for the pelvic tilt, all trunk movements including rotations, forward bendings, and side flexions done in sitting. These exercises would strengthen the spine at the same time.

SCOLIOSIS

By scoliosis a lateral curving and rotating of the spine is meant. Unlike the exaggerated normal curves which exist in lordosis and kyphosis the curves of scoliosis are quite abnormal. A postural scoliosis where the structures of the spine have not yet altered can be corrected, but maintenance of the correct posture takes much time and practice to accomplish for long periods. If the postural scoliosis is not treated, it will eventually become permanent and changes in the muscles, ligaments, bones, and joints will inevitably take place. A postural curve consists of a single curve of the spine in one direction only in any one of the three mobile regions of the spine. That is in the cervical or thoracic or lumbar regions. Sometimes the whole spine is involved in a long 'C' curve. When the 'C' curve becomes permanent very often other compensatory curves appear in the rest of the spine in different directions, so that an 'S' curve may appear or even three and sometimes four curves can be seen in the spine. The latter are rare and are very often caused as a result of some other existing deformity. Postural curves, as the name implies, are very often the result of repeated bad postural habits. *The aim in treating a postural scoliosis* would be to correct the general posture. The muscles maintaining the correct posture are the muscles of the head and neck, the extensors of the back, the abdominal muscles, extensors of hip and knee, and small muscles of the feet. Static contractions would be given to these muscles in lying, sitting, and standing, and the client would be encouraged to maintain a good posture whilst performing added arm, head, and trunk exercises. More difficult exercises involving balance and co-ordination would finally be taught. It is the holding of a good posture during the exercise which is of value and not the exercise itself.

WINGED SCAPULA

This is a condition in which the vertebral border and inferior angle of the scapula protrudes backwards away from the ribs when the arm is lifted forwards to shoulder level. The client will be unable to punch the arm forward or perform forward pushing movements or lift the arm above shoulder level. It is often due to a weakness of the serratus anterior.

EXERCISES FOR WINGED SCAPULA

Position: sitting.

1. Lift both arms forwards to shoulder level. The client will find this difficult.
2. Pushing and punching forwards with the hands against the resistance of the therapist's hands.

Position: standing.

1. Place one hand on a wall and push forwards. Change and push with the other.
2. Both arms swing forwards, backwards, forwards, upwards, and circle backwards, down and round.
3. Both arms lift forwards to shoulder level, stretch sideways to shoulder level, lift up by the side of the head, and lower forwards and down to the sides.
4. Lean forwards onto a wall supporting body with hands against the wall, arms bent. Push arms straight and body upright, slowly lower onto the wall again (a modified version of press-ups).
5. All swinging movements of the arms at the shoulder joint.

WEAK ABDOMINAL MUSCLES AND VISCEROPTOSIS

Visceroptosis is a condition in which the abdominal and pelvic organs are very often displaced downwards. It is commonly caused through over-stretched and weakened abdominal muscles. The abdominal muscles act in several ways. They flex the spine bending the trunk forwards, or draw the pelvis and legs upwards if the thorax is fixed. Together with the back muscles, the muscles of the one side flex the spine and trunk to the same side, and the obliquus muscles rotate the spine and trunk round. They also assist respiration in forced expiration and the support of the abdominal contents depends greatly on their muscle tone, together with the internal muscles of the pelvic floor. These pelvic floor muscles help with excretion, and support the contents of the pelvis and abdomen from below the pelvis like a sling preventing them from dropping out.

Very often certain body types are prone to weakness of these muscles although child-bearing, abdominal operations, poor posture, obesity, nervousness, or lack of sufficient exercise are among some of the contributory causes for weakened abdominal muscles. It is the strengthening of these abdominal muscles which is the prime concern of the beauty therapist, but it is wise to find out the cause for their weakness before commencing treatment. Visceroptosis can be a condition affecting any age and can vary in degree. Obviously not all those whose abdominal muscles are weak suffer from visceroptosis but eventually some degree or other of it may occur as a result of poor muscular tone in this area. Prevention is better than cure, and strong abdominal muscles help to avoid complications that may or may not arise.

Signs and symptoms: The client who has weakened abdominal muscles may appear to have a prominent and bulging abdomen. She may tell the beauty therapist that she has dragging sensations, constipation, or attacks of intense pain. Very often she is nervous and highly excitable. If the therapist suspects any medical condition exists whatsoever or encounters untoward signs and symptoms, she should first check with the doctor before attempting any corrective treatment. However, if the client has a severe condition of visceroptosis, it is doubtful that she would have found her way to the beauty therapist in the first place. What the beauty therapist is basically treating is the weakened abdominal muscles. The following selection of exercises are suitable for clients with a weak stretched abdominal wall. They will also help to mobilize the spine. Progression from lying into standing would be advisable in these cases. They should be done slowly, gently, and with complete control.

EXERCISES FOR WEAK ABDOMINAL MUSCLES

Position: crook lying.

1. Press the small of the back down onto the bed pulling in the abdominal muscles.
2. Bend both knees gently over to the right keeping the feet on the floor, then slowly over to the left.
3. Sideways bend to slide right arm down to grasp right ankle, repeat sliding left hand to grasp left ankle.
4. Lift head and shoulders off the bed and lie back again.
5. Stretch arms out sideways to shoulder level, reach over with the right hand to touch the left hand keeping the hips flat on the bed. Change with left hand over the right hand.
6. Bend the right knee up onto the chest and change positions with the left.
7. Press the knees and thighs together squeezing the gluteal muscles (buttocks) tightly, just lifting the hips off the bed (pelvic floor muscles are tightened here).

Position: long sitting.

1. Bend over to touch toes with both hands.
2. Place feet apart, stretch over to grasp right ankle with left hand and then change to grasp left ankle with right hand.
3. Fingertips on the shoulders, sideways bend to the right and then to the left.
4. Raise arms sideways to shoulder level, turn trunk round to the right and then to the left.

Position: sitting.

1. Fold arms across the chest, stand up.
2. Lift right knee upwards, change and lift left knee upwards.
3. Knees apart, place fingertips on shoulders, stretch over to touch right knee with left elbow, change to touch left knee with right elbow.
4. Turn trunk to look over left shoulder and then over right shoulder.

5. Cross right leg over the left, squeeze the thighs together at the top, tighten the seat muscles, and pull in the abdominal muscles. Change over legs and repeat these contractions to the other side (pelvic floor static contractions; the therapist must see that the client does not hold her breath).

Position: stride standing.

1. Swing arms round from side to side, keeping hips facing forwards.
2. Slide right arm sideways down right thigh to back of the knee with a push, at the same time stretch the left arm sideways over the head. Change to bend to the opposite side pushing down on the left side with the right arm over the right side of the head.
3. Stand with one leg in front of the other and apart, lean forwards, and twist the trunk and arms from side to side as though using a scythe. Change position of legs and repeat the action.

SOME VERY STRONG ABDOMINAL EXERCISES

Position: lying.

1. Bend legs on to the abdomen, stretch legs in the air straight, and lower straight to the ground (uses abdominal muscles eccentrically and as extensors of the spine and hips).
2. Lift both legs straight in the air (uses abdominal muscles concentrically in middle and inner range, and as flexors of hips and spine).
3. Place both hands behind the head and sit up bending over to touch straight knees with head (uses abdominal muscles concentrically origin and insertion reversed, also stretches hamstrings).
4. Cross ankles over and press knees, insides of thighs, gluteal muscles at the same time. Change over legs and repeat.

Position: hanging.

1. Bend both knees onto chest, bend them over to the right side and then round to the left rotating at the waist and spine.

2. Bend knees onto chest, stretch legs out straight in front of the body, and lower slowly down.
3. Swing both legs at waist and spine sideways to the right and then to the left.
4. Lift both straight legs forwards and upwards.

Exercise, Massage, and Obesity

Many hundreds and thousands of men and women all over the world are more weight- and figure-conscious than ever before. Why do they come to the beauty salons, health farms, and sauna baths to mention but a few of the places where advice and help in figure correction can be found? There are many reasons. Perhaps one may be some sudden spring sunshine and realization that summer holidays and revealing bikinis are not too far around the corner. Perhaps another is in preparation for winter sports, or to be able to wear a new dress with ease that now feels too tight, or to boost up the confidence of a teenager who feels that success in dating boy friends might be hers at last if her figure is righted. Sometimes women who are experiencing the menopause feel that their youth and looks have ebbed away, and they need the reassurance that beauty therapy can give, by helping them to do something positive about it. For some men who seek physical fitness, their motives lie in the need to be successful with women, which they feel only comes with looks, health, and beauty. Mental health and physical health go hand in hand, and everyone realizes that being overweight is hazardous and unhealthy for the heart and body. This is probably the main reason for doing something about it by asking the expert. Looking better makes one feel better, although the old saying that 'beauty is in the eye of the beholder' stands very true. Not everyone cares or is even interested in trying to alter their physical appearance, and sometimes this careless attitude is deliberately cultivated. It really does not matter what the basic reason is for slimming or changing shape; the fact remains that most people, if given a chance to improve their figure and size by the wave of a magic wand would take it, and do so. The beauty therapist must respect whatever good reasons the client has, no matter how trivial they may seem, that bring her to seek professional advice and help which will build up the confidence and ego of the client.

TYPES OF OBESITY

Before treating obesity it is as well to understand the different types that there are.

1. There is the type of obesity which could be called *hereditary*. This is the kind where no treatment seems to be of permanent benefit. When asked it will be discovered that the client's mother and grandmother were fat, and that indeed many members of the family tended towards obesity.
2. Another kind of obesity is attributed to the malfunctioning of the *glandular* system. For example, an under-secretion of the thyroid gland would result in the carbohydrates and fats being stored as body fat due to faulty metabolism. Fat, too, may be stored in the body during the menopause when the hormone balance is disturbed. This kind of fat, that is not oxidized properly nor broken down sufficiently in the process of digestion, seems to settle round the abdomen, hips, and thighs. Middle-aged spread refers to these areas and the change of life between forty and fifty.
3. The most common reason for being overweight is that caused by *overeating*. This can take the form of generally eating too much, excess eating of the wrong kinds of foods, or an unbalanced diet coupled with insufficient exercise. These are the cases which can be treated most successfully. Very often it is the middle-aged person who has the means to indulge in richer foods, heavier drinking, and a more sedentary life, who finds weight is becoming a problem. However, these days it seems that carrying only one or two extra pounds of weight on the body constitutes a case for treatment. So the beauty therapist is faced with the task of prescribing and advising either general or localized treatments for all, no matter how slim or what age or sex.

TREATMENT

Treatment must only be undertaken after first having checked with the doctor to ascertain the cause, and to confirm that the general health of the client is good. He will be able to prescribe a suitable diet which will probably cut down on starchy foods, sugars, and fats. There are many excellent diets some of which forbid certain foods entirely; others advocate the eating of more of one kind than another. The therapist should be able to supply the kind of diet to fit the case if required to do so. Crash diets are only advisable for a short period of time, and very often a drastic weight loss in a few days can result in making the client look haggard. A slow steady loss over a period of weeks is healthier, better, and more advisable.

It has been well established that the ideal form of treatment for obesity is by a combination of *diet, massage,* and *exercise,* and even then there can be no guarantee. If the weight is to be reduced at all substantially then the full co-operation of the client is the most important factor of all. She must adhere strictly to the diet, not be allowed to expect too much from the massage, and be prepared to practise the exercises faithfully, which will help to oxidize and burn up the fatty deposits.

If massage is to be used in conjunction with the diet and exercise programme, the massage should be interspersed between the exercises, and should treat only those areas where excess fat may be found. For very obese clients a general massage could be given followed by a general scheme of rigorous exercises. In most people the fatty deposits are usually found on the back of the neck and shoulders, back of the upper arms, round the sides of the thorax, waist, abdomen, hips, thighs, and buttocks.

The massage must be very vigorous to these areas to have any effect. It is often said that the only person who loses weight by massage is the masseuse, which proves the point that the therapist has to work hard in order to crush the fat by massage.

Consideration for the client is important, and if she is grossly overweight then exercises in the lying or sitting position could be more suitable until there has been a considerable weight loss, by which time the muscles would be improved in tone. Otherwise exercises in all positions would be given. Much encouragement must be given to the client to enable her to persevere, and she should be weighed and measured once a week. Even the smallest weight loss must be recorded and made known to the client, for encouragement to continue. Home exercises must be stressed, but they should be kept to a minimum and fairly simple.

FIGURE CORRECTION EXERCISES

Here are some good figure correction exercises for the beauty therapist to teach the client which should help to trim the fatty trouble spots and firm the body contours. They can be divided into two groups. The first group consists of *mobility* exercises to be repeated several times and with a quick loose rhythm along the lines described earlier in the chapter. These will not only loosen and warm up the parts but will tone the muscles and help to break down the fat at the same time. The second group are *strengthening* exercises which will tone and build up the muscles also firming up the lines. Breathing exercises, relaxation, and postural correction should punctuate both the general and localized schemes of exercises. The following exercises can be used together with all the other exercises described in devising general keep-fit schemes.

MOBILITY EXERCISES

TROUBLE SPOT ONE

Back of the upper arms and shoulders.

Position: standing or sitting.

Main muscles in action: triceps.

1. Inwardly rotate both arms, raising them sideways to shoulder level so that the palms of the hands are facing down and the backs of the elbows uppermost; hold this position; now bend and stretch the elbows quickly.
2. Stretch arms straight up by the side of the head with palms

facing, holding this position; now bend and stretch the arms alternately and quickly, keeping the elbows pointing up in the air as elbows bend.

3. Stretch arms sideways to shoulder level, palms facing forwards; hold this position; now bend elbows, touch shoulders with fingertips, and straighten elbows pulling arms as far back as possible at the same time.

TROUBLE SPOT TWO

Shoulder and back of neck region.

Position: standing.

Main muscles in action: upper fibres of trapezius, deep neck muscles, rhomboids, and latissimus dorsi.

1. Swing both arms backwards, forwards, backwards, and then forwards and circling round in large circles.
2. Drop head forwards chin onto chest and pull the head backwards and up, keeping the chin tucked in, and slowly bend the neck backwards to look up in the air.
3. Lean forwards from the hips, keeping the back straight and allowing the arms to hang freely in front of the body; hold this position; now swing the arms across the body, then out sideways, then again across the body in front of the face, standing up straight to circle them up, outwards, and down, and across into the original position.

TROUBLE SPOT THREE

Front of neck, chest, and jaw line.

Position: sitting or standing.

Main muscles in action: platysma, masseter (muscle of mastication) sterno-mastoid, deep muscles on front of vertebrae.

1. Clench and unclench teeth and jaw.
2. Depress the angles of the mouth downwards and sideways in an expression of horror, tightening the skin under the jawline, front of neck, and across the chest.

3. Turn head to left, right, up, and down. Bend right ear onto right shoulder; bend left ear onto left shoulder. Circle head round in one direction then the other.
4. Press head and neck backwards, tucking in the chin, pushing up top of the head, straightening the cervical spine.

TROUBLE SPOT FOUR

Scapular, middle and upper back region.

Position: standing or sitting.

Main muscles in action: rotators, elevators, adductors, and depressors of scapulae. In- and outward rotators of shoulder joint.

1. Shrug shoulders tightly up and down.
2. Pull shoulder blades backwards and together.
3. Place one hand behind the neck and one behind the waist with a swing; quickly change positions.

TROUBLE SPOT FIVE

Chest wall, midriff, and waist.

Position: stride standing or sitting.

Main muscles in action: abdominal muscles, back muscles.

1. Place fingertips on the shoulder; hold this position; now bend sideways with a bounce to the right, up and over with a bounce to the left side.
2. Stretch both arms above the head and bend as far back as possible; hold this position; now bend over to touch the toes with each hand and with a bounce between each bend and stretch.
3. Bend trunk over and touch left foot with right hand; stretch up and twist trunk round to the right, raising the right arm sideways to shoulder level stretching it back as far as possible and turning the head to the right at the same time. Repeat to the other side.
4. Raise arms sideways to shoulder level; hold this position; now twist the trunk around from side to side as far as possible to

the right and left as far as possible, keeping the hips facing forwards as the trunk rotates.

5. Stretch arms above head; hold this position; now swing the arms and trunk downwards between the legs, and upwards in large movements.

TROUBLE SPOT SIX

Bust.

Position: standing or sitting.

Main muscles in action: pectorals, platysma.

1. Stretch head back to look in the air; depress the angles of the mouth and lower jaw as hard as possible in horror expression. Platysma tightens to apex of shoulders and across chest, lifting up the bosom.
2. Raise the arms forwards to shoulder level, fold the forearms across the chest right hand encircling left wrist and left hand encircling right wrist. Push up the skin on the forearms as though trying to push up the sleeves of a dress.
3. Raise arms to shoulder level; grasp right arm upper with left hand, and the left upper arm with right hand across in front of the chest; hold this position; push each arm firmly with opposite hand as though to force them away. Feel the breasts jerk upwards as the pectorals tighten.
4. Correction of posture and particularly in pushing up the crown of the head high and back, with chin tucked in, does much to improve the bust line.

TROUBLE SPOT SEVEN

Waist and abdomen.

Position: lying.

Main muscles in action: abdominal.

1. Bend both knees with feet on the floor, stretch arms sideways on the floor to shoulder level palms facing down; hold this

position; now bend right arm over to the left repeating quickly to the opposite sides.

2. Bend knees, hold this position; now sit up quickly and lie down again.

3. Place legs apart, hold this position; now sit up quickly reaching over to touch left foot with right hand, lie down and quickly repeat with the other hand to opposite foot.

4. Tighten and straighten right leg and knee, pull up toes to point to the ceiling, hold this position; now shorten the right leg on the floor by pulling it up and in from the right waist region as hard as possible, repeat with the other leg.

TROUBLE SPOT EIGHT

Hips, buttocks, and tops of thighs.

Position: standing.

Main muscles in action: gluteal muscles, hip extensors.

1. Hold sideways onto a support and swing right leg backwards and forwards as far as possible allowing knee to bend on backwards swing. Repeat with other leg.

2. Jump feet apart and together with small rebounds between each jump, keeping trunk upright.

Position: prone lying.

1. Keeping knee bent lift the right leg backwards quickly changing with the left leg.

Position: lying.

1. Bend knees, feet flat on the floor, hold this position; lift hips upwards and downwards quickly squeezing seat muscles tightly together as the trunk is raised in a straight line with thighs.

TROUBLE SPOT NINE

Thighs and hips.

Position: standing.

Main muscles in action: abductors, hamstrings, quadriceps, adductors, and gluteals.

1. Lift right knee up as high as possible; change with the left knee quickly until running on the spot. Knees lifted high throughout.

Position: side lying.

1. Make sure that the body is in a straight line with trunk, one leg on top of the other; lift top leg sideways to the body up and down quickly.
2. Swing top leg backwards and forwards allowing knee to bend and stretch with the swing.
3. Circle top leg round moving it forwards sideways and up, backwards down and round again in large circles, keeping the knee straight and foot pulled up.
4. Change over to the opposite side and repeat the above exercises with the other leg.

TROUBLE SPOT TEN

Calves, ankles, and feet.

Position: sitting.

Main muscles in action: anterior and posterior tibial muscles, intrinsic muscles, of the feet.

1. Tuck feet slightly under the knees but keep them flat out on the floor, hold this position; now raise heel of right foot, change quickly with the left foot stretching the ankles as far as possible.
2. Stretch the legs and feet out in front resting on the heels, hold this position; now pull up the toes and ankles of the right foot and quickly change with the left.
3. Keep legs and feet stretched out in front on heels, hold the position; now turn soles of feet in to face each other and pull up the toes and ankles at the same time, now stretch the toes down again turning the soles of the feet out and away from each other.

4. Position as above.

    Circle toes round and round from the ankles first one way and then the other.

5. Still with feet stretched out on to the heels again, pull up the toes and ankles, hold this position; now bend over the toes and stretch them back again quickly. Try to keep the toes straight and prevent them from clawing over.

6. Place feet flat on the floor a little apart, hold this position; now grip the floor firmly with the toes trying to press them into it but keeping them quite straight and extended. They should shorten and lift the arches of the feet higher.

STRENGTHENING EXERCISES

TROUBLE SPOT ONE

Back of arms.

Position: prone lying.

1. Press-ups, lifting body off the floor in a straight line by means of pushing down on the hands and straightening the elbows. Important to see that hands are placed underneath the shoulder joint.

Position: standing.

1. Press the back of the slightly flexed forearm against a wall trying to straighten the elbow.

2. Stand between a doorway, arms at shoulder level, elbows flexed with the dorsum of the hands against the uprights, hold this position; now push the back of the hands as hard as possible as though trying to push the doorposts out.

TROUBLE SPOT TWO

Shoulder girdle, head, and neck.

Position: hanging.

1. With hands gripping the bar at not less than shoulder width apart, pull the weight of the body as far upwards as possible slowly.

2. Lift head and neck backwards.

Position: prone lying.

1. Place hands underneath forehead with elbows flexed and bent, hold this position: now lift head, shoulders, hands, and elbows backwards off the floor as far as possible.
2. Stretch both arms up by the side of the head along the floor or bed hold this position; now lift straight arms, head, neck, and shoulders as far backwards as possible.
3. Keep arms stretched above head; lift one arm and head backwards off the floor, change with the other without touching the floor between each arm lift.

TROUBLE SPOT THREE

Front of neck.

Position: lying.

1. Lift head off the floor, hold, and lower.
2. Lift head off the floor turn it to the right and then to the left.
3. Place hands with elbows bent on forehead hold this position: now lift head, hands, and arms off the floor.

TROUBLE SPOT FOUR

Upper back region.

Position: prone lying.

1. Place hands, with elbows flexed, underneath forehead; lift head, shoulders, arms, and hands backwards off the floor; hold this position; now turn trunk to the right, then to the left as though to look over right and left shoulders respectively.
2. Place arms sideways to shoulder level along the floor; hold this position; now lift backwards arms, head, and neck, as far as possible, pulling shoulder blades together.
3. Place hands under the forehead with elbows flexed, lift head, shoulders, elbows, and hands backwards off the floor; hold this position; now bend the trunk sideways down to the right side, and then sideways down to the left side.

TROUBLE SPOT FIVE

Chest wall, midriff, and waist.

Position: lying.

1. Hold onto a support with hands if necessary; now lift the right leg up off the floor as high as possible; lower but not quite to the ground; change with the left leg slowly in a scissor action.
2. Stretch arms at shoulder-width apart in the air in front of the face; hold this position; now keeping the arms stretched in the air, sit up (they should now be by the side of the head); lie down again.
3. Stretch legs apart and place hand behind head hold this position; now sit up and bend over to touch right knee with left elbow; lie down and sit up again, touching left knee with right elbow.
4. Bend knees, place hands on front of forehead, hold this position; now sit up and then twist the body slowly round to the right and then slowly to the left.

TROUBLE SPOT SIX

Bust.

Position: lying.

1. Stretch arms sideways along the floor to shoulder level; lift them to stretch up into the air in front of the face, and lower them back by the sides of the head on the floor; lower them down by the sides again.
2. Place arms sideways to shoulder level and lift arms forwards to cross in front of the face, touching back of left shoulder with right hand and right shoulder with left hand.
3. Hold a weight in each hand tightly and lift arms forwards to shoulder level from the sides of the body, from the sides of the head, and from abduction sideways at shoulder level.

TROUBLE SPOT SEVEN

Waist and abdomen.

Position: lying.

All strong abdominal exercises described under the section dealing with visceroptosis and weak abdominal muscles.

Extra exercises would include bicycling legs round in the air, bending knees onto the chest and stretching them over from side to side from the waist, both exercises in the lying position. Strengthening exercises from trouble spot five.

TROUBLE SPOT EIGHT

Hips, buttocks, and tops of thighs.

Position: prone lying.

1. Lie with trunk only on the bed and legs over the edge down on the floor; grip the bed firmly with the arms above the head; hold this position; now lift back the right leg off the floor slowly, then change with the left, then lift back both legs together off the floor till they are in a straight line with the trunk.

Position: prone kneeling.

1. Bend right knee up to the chest, stretch back straightening leg in the air, in line with the body; repeat with the left leg.
2. Stretch right leg sideways on the floor, lift it backwards in the air, bring it into line with the body, still stretched backwards in the air, bend it down to original position, and repeat with left leg.

Position: kneeling.

1. Sit back on heels, place hands behind neck, and sit up straight to lift trunk off heels in straight line with thighs.

Position: prone lying.

1. Lie with trunk over the edge of bed, hands behind neck. Client will need supporting and holding across legs to stop her toppling forwards, hold this position; now lift trunk backwards and upwards as far as possible (very strong exercise for gluteals and back muscles).

TROUBLE SPOT NINE

Thighs and hips.

Position: side lying.

1. Lie on right side with legs in a straight line with body. Lift the right leg with the weight of the left leg on it up in the air, and repeat on the other side with the left leg. This exercises the adductor muscles of the thigh and also the waist muscles may come strongly into action.
2. Lie on the right side; lift the straight left leg sideways and upwards in the air. This uses the abductors of the leg.

Position: sitting on the floor.

1. Cross the legs and place the right hand on the right knee, left hand on the left knee hold this position; press both hands down, and now try to bring knees upwards and together. This is for the inner side of the thigh.
2. Bend knees into a crook position, stretch both legs out in front, and then draw body up to legs bending the knees into the crook position again using the back of the thigh muscles.

Position: kneeling.

1. Sit back on heels keeping body in straight line, try to pull up into kneeling again using inner thigh muscles.

Position: standing.

1. Hold onto a support, stretch up on to tiptoes, bend knees fully and bounce slowly up and down in the knees bent position, for quadriceps.

Position: prone lying.

1. Tuck toes underneath on floor with ankle in dorsiflexion, brace back the knee tightly so the leg is straight; hold this position; now lift straight leg backwards just off the floor; using back of hip and thigh muscles.

TROUBLE SPOT TEN

Calves, ankles, and feet.

Position: standing.

1. Stretch right ankle up on to ball of feet, slowly change with left foot.
2. Walk forwards fifty paces slowly on toes with ankles stretched, walk fifty paces normally.
3. Walk forwards fifty paces on heels, walk fifty paces normally.
4. Grip floor with toes keeping them straight, lifting the arches on the inside border of the feet.

N.B. Whilst giving any exercise the therapist should not forget to correct the client's posture throughout each exercise and to make sure that the client is breathing normally. The client must be reminded that Rome was not built in a day, and that to expect any significant change or result in less than two or three months would be wishful thinking, especially if she is not prepared to practise her exercises at home.

II. *Breathing and Relaxation*

The importance of correct breathing for health and beauty is underestimated. It is not quite as automatic as most people imagine. All the systems and tissues of the body require for their functioning and for body metabolism an ample supply of oxygen. This is ensured and promoted by the correct gaseous interchange which takes place in the lungs through respiration. Resistance to infection is increased when the lungs are utilized thoroughly, maintaining and improving their elasticity and strength. If all the lung tissue is exercised frequently their secretions are less likely to stagnate and accumulate. Coughs and colds will be few and far between. Posture is improved with correct breathing; the mind becomes more active and alert, nerves are calmed by deep breathing, circulation is quickened, eyes are bright and clear, fat is oxidized and muscles are fed. The secret of correct breathing can control the speaking voice and the movements of the body, both of which are vital aides to being beautiful. Correct breathing assists relaxation, even in childbirth.

Mechanics of Respiration

The air enters the body via the nose where it is filtered and warmed before it passes into the lungs. The lungs are two balloon-like structures each with an upper, middle, and lower region or lobe, joined together at the top into one central passage known as the trachea. This links up to the back of the mouth and nose.

Respiration can be divided into two parts, namely inspiration, when the air is drawn into the body, and expiration, when the air is expelled.

Inspiration involves the contraction of the diaphragm, intercostal and other respiratory muscles which enlarge the thorax in several directions. When the diaphragm contracts, it descends and expands, pushing out the abdomen. The rib cage is also pulled out vertically like a concertina. As the intercostal and other muscles contract they cause the ribs to be elevated laterally and antero-posteriorly like the lifting of a bucket handle, or the opening of venetian blinds. When the contractions take place the air rushes into all sections of the lungs. If the diaphragm is not used properly then the lower regions of the lungs will not be ventilated or expanded and will become neglected. Breathing is shallower and is restricted to the upper part of the chest. A common fault on inspiration is to pull in the abdomen, which prevents the diaphragm from functioning correctly, limiting the breathing capacity.

Expiration normally involves a mere relaxation of all the respiratory muscles, returning the thorax to its original size. However, when the expiration is forced, the abdominal muscles contract and are retracted, flattening and even hollowing the abdomen; the diaphragm is pushed upwards, and the chest hollows as the sternum and lower ribs are pulled down in an effort to expel the maximum amount of air from the lungs. Breathing becomes very deep.

Some Important Points

Breathing exercises can be practised in all positions, so that whatever exercise is being carried out and in whichever position, a breathing exercise can and should always be incorporated. The breathing exercise can be purely for breathing, or for a combination of exercise and breathing. In this way the client is prevented from holding her breath, a maximum oxygen supply to the working muscles is ensured, she can learn the difference between tension and relaxation in the muscles, and, when breathing is combined with arm and trunk exercises, the whole respiratory system is used to full advantage. However, the breathing should be in the client's own time, but when combining the two it is generally carried out according to the therapist's instructions for guidance. Interspersing pure breathing in an exercise scheme has its advantages also. This method provides a useful resting point in which the client can relax and recoup her energy, regaining her normal rhythm of breathing after a particularly strenuous bout of exercises. If she is placed in the lying position for the exercises, the knees should be bent as in crook lying to relax the abdominal muscles. After the initial instruction and correction of the right way in which to breathe, she shou'd be allowed to breathe in and out in her own time. Too much deep breathing can cause light-headedness, dizziness, and even fainting, especially if there is little muscle work taking place in the body. Restricting each exercise to three times, and to a maximum of three exercises at a time to be given consecutively, minimizes this temporary effect. In a general keep-fit scheme of exercises, both pure breathing and breathing combined with an exercise can be included. This helps to add interest and vary the exercises. Because even the fittest client may feel a little light-headed after too much deep breathing, it is as well to ask her from time to time if she feels all right. Before the breathing exercises are begun, the client should empty the air out of the lungs by blowing out first.

THREE KINDS OF BREATHING

Apical uses the upper lobe of the lungs and is shallow, high, and rapid. High temperatures, illness, fear, excitement, anger, respiratory diseases, such as bronchitis or asthma, are some precursors to this kind of breathing. Sometimes athletes use it for a quick intake of oxygen, and apical breathing takes place during childbirth whilst the diaphragm muscle helps to fix the thorax and push the baby out of the birth canal.

Lateral costal uses the upper and middle lobes of the lungs. It is deeper and slower than apical breathing and it is this kind of breathing that many people use unwittingly most of the time, together with apical.

Diaphragmatic uses the upper, middle, and lower lobes of the lungs. It is deep and calm and should be used whenever possible at all times.

All three kinds of breathing exercises should be explained and taught to the client so that a complete overall picture of the breathing mechanism is obtained. However, in health and beauty, it is only the diaphragmatic breathing which is emphasized and practised. This guarantees full and correct use of the normal healthy respiratory system.

TECHNIQUE

APICAL BREATHING

Position: stride standing.

1. Place hands flat either side of chest just below clavicles; blow out.
2. Take a short breath in through the nose, pushing up the upper part of the chest under the hands, slightly lifting the shoulders.
3. To the short sharp sound of 'Sh', blow out the air through the mouth. The client will hear the air being expelled and feel the chest relaxing.
4. Repeat this breathing rapidly no more than three times as explained previously. The client will feel the chest lifting up and down.

LATERAL COSTAL BREATHING

Position: stride standing.

1. Place the hands flat on either side of the chest wall below the axillae and above the waist. Blow out.
2. Take a deeper breath in through the nose keeping the upper part of the chest and shoulders down and relaxed, pushing out the sides of the ribs. She will feel this expansion sideways with her hands.
3. To the sound of 'Ha' blow out the air through the mouth.

The client will feel the ribs concertina down and she can hear the air being blown out. It will be a longer respiration than apical breathing.

4. Repeat the breathing in the client's own time, emphasizing the expiration.

DIAPHRAGMATIC BREATHING

Position: stride standing.

1. Place the flat hand either side and across the front lower ribs. The fingertips should be touching each other just below the xiphoid process of the sternum. Blow out.
2. Take a long deep breath in through the nose, pushing up the hands in front, and the ribs out at the sides. If the diaphragm muscle is being used properly, the fingers will be parted in front on expansion of the thorax. This can be felt with the hands guiding and encouraging the client to greater effort.
3. To the sound of 'S' blow out the air for as long as possible, by pulling in the abdominal muscles as hard as possible at the same time. The client will hear the air being expired, feel the rib cage descending, fingers coming together again, and the abdomen pulling in.
4. The breathing is repeated in the client's own time.

RELAXED BREATHING

The normal natural rhythm of relaxed diaphragmatic breathing with a gentle rise and fall of the abdominal muscles on breathing in and out respectively is soon acquired. There should be no exaggerated heaving of the chest and shoulders. The air has to pass through the upper and middle regions when the lower lobes are being used as in the relaxed diaphragmatic breathing. With relaxed breathing the client should be instructed to breathe in and out of the nose.

SOME GENERAL EXERCISES COMBINED WITH DEEP DIAPHRAGMATIC BREATHING

Remember: breathe in through the nose, blow out through the mouth.

Position: stride standing.

1. Lift both arms sideways and up into elevation by the side of the head taking a deep breath in at the same time. When maximum inspiration is obtained, slowly blow the air out of the mouth, lowering the arms at a steady rate to the sides at the same time.
2. Place the fingertips on the shoulders, circle the elbows round beginning by lifting them forwards and upwards to point in the air, sideways and down. As they are lifted forwards and up, a deep long breath in should be taken; as they lower down sideways the air should be blown out of the mouth.
3. Bend the trunk sideways sliding the right arm down the right leg blowing out at the same time. Stretch the trunk upright to the middle again, breathing in. Bend over to the left side blowing out and up to the middle, breathing in.

Position: stride sitting.

1. Bend over to touch the floor between the feet, blowing out. Slowly sit up lifting arms above the head and breathing in deeply. Bend over to touch floor again breathing out.
2. Place fingertips on shoulders and twist over to touch right knee with left elbow, blowing out. Stretch upright to middle, breathing in. Twist over to touch left knee with right elbow, blowing out; sit up, breathe in.

Position: prone lying.

1. Place hands under forehead, lift head, shoulder, arms, and hands backwards off the floor or bed, breathing in. Lower down, blowing out.
2. Lift both legs, head, and shoulder backwards, breathing in; lower down, blowing out.

Position: crook lying.

1. Lift trunk and bottom upwards, tightening gluteal muscles, till body is in a straight line with the thighs; breathe in at the same time, lower hips, blowing out.
2. Bend both knees over to the right to touch the floor, blowing

out. Bring them back to the middle, breathing in deeply. Bend them over to the left blowing out; to the middle, breathing in.

Relaxation

Relaxation can be defined as the release of tension in the mind and body, and is a desirable state which is pursued by everyone in some form or other. It has long since been agreed by the medical profession that tension of the mind can cause muscle tension, disease, illness, pain, and even proneness to accidents. These in turn can cause relaxation to be impossible, so creating a vicious circle. The beauty therapist knows and often sees the havoc that can be played in the face and in the general posture, from a mind racked by problems and tensions, or aches and pains, from which there seems to be no respite. Mental and physical tension cannot be easily separated, but one thing is for sure and this is, that a relaxed mind is housed in a relaxed and healthy body, and a relaxed and healthy body relates closely to a relaxed and healthy mind.

WHY RELAX?

Relaxation of the muscles of the body is used sometimes to enable them to be spurred on to greater physical efforts. Sometimes it is used to block out mental thoughts as a means to inducing sleep. Although it is said by certain authorities that sleep and total relaxation are not synonymous, for even during sleep dreams occur and some muscles maintain a strong degree of tone, yet usually most of the muscles are relaxed in sleep, and dreaming is a normal phenomenon. However, to be able to drift into a deep relaxed sleep and wake up feeling vitally alive and refreshed, instead of tossing and turning half the night, sleeping lightly, and waking up as though never having been to bed at all, is for many an enviable state.

Recreation, amusements, television, sports and hobbies, drugs, alcohol, sex, and holidays are but a few of the means used as vital pathways to escape from the cares of life and work. They are mostly applied entirely to the mind and bring with them their own special brand of side effects which, if not harmful, can in turn be tension-provoking, so that even mental relaxation is only partially achieved. A change is not always as good as a rest.

PHILOSOPHY

Relaxation of the mind and body can become a philosophy and a way of life to be learned, being of great value to the individual. Ridding the body of unconscious mental and physical tension means that the mind can take it easy and refuse to become unnecessarily excited. Living slows down to a steady rate, instead of a constant rush with never enough days in the week. Holidays can be taken instead of being needed. Learning to relax for this aim is an art which needs to be practised in order to be mastered. Like an elusive pimpernel, relaxation may take weeks to accomplish. When once having acquired the ability to relax by whatever method, it can be utilized as a pacemaker for two or three minutes at a time whenever pressures begin to crowd in throughout the hustling rush and bustle of a busy day.

WHEN TO PRACTISE

The best time to learn how to relax is before going to sleep at night. For those who suffer from insomnia, relaxation can be a means of luring sleep. It has already been stressed that it must be practised regularly to be perfected and it would be best to advise the client to retire to bed half an hour earlier than usual to specifically practise the art of relaxation.

AIDS TO RELAXATION

A brisk walk before retiring is recommended as a preliminary to relaxation and sleep. It requires little effort depending entirely on available time and personal strength. Loose rhythmic movements of the arms and legs should be adopted which will produce a pleasant warm tired sensation and gentle muscular fatigue.

Active exercises are another preliminary which would prove to be helpful and conducive to relaxation. They need only take ten minutes. Each movement should be done five times or until slight fatigue is felt in the working muscles.

The sequence of exercises is as follows:

1. *Foot, ankle, and toe* movements such as bouncing up and down on toes with heels raised.
2. *Knee* movements lifting first one knee up in the air and then the other.
3. *Hip* backward and forward swinging and then circling the whole leg round, holding on to a support.
4. *Wrist, hand, and finger* movements such as quick fist and hand flapping.
5. *Trunk* forward bending and circling round in both directions to mobilize the spine.
6. *Elbow* movements involving bending and stretching elbows alternately by placing fingertips on shoulders from the sides of the body quickly.
7. *Shoulder* and whole arm swinging round in circles.
8. *Shoulder girdle* shrugging up and down and pulling back shoulder blades.
9. *Neck and cervical spine* movements consisting of head turning and circling.
10. *Scalp* movement consisting of linking fingers together across the top of the scalp and sliding them forwards and backwards at the same time as flexing and extending the neck.
11. *Brisk rub-down* all over the body with the palmar surface of the hands on the skin to stimulate the superficial circulation and leave a warm sense of glowing.

At first during the practising period avoid competitive games as they tend to leave the mind in a highly active state which will hinder relaxation.

Warmth by taking a hot bath or a warm drink is important, for muscles cannot relax if they are cold.

Ventilation is essential, without producing a draught, to ensure an ample supply of fresh air. Stuffiness is unhealthy although the oxygen requirements are considerably less when the body is at rest.

Disturbance and noise should be avoided as much as possible; the client should ask her family to co-operate in this matter.

Darkness in the room will help to cut out visual impulses for, even though the eyes may be closed, a bright light can still penetrate through the eyelids.

Comfort by means of pillows and a well-sprung mattress can make relaxation and sleep more of a certainty. The client should not be wearing tight restricting clothes. She should adopt her most comfortable sleeping position and use sufficient pillows for her maximum comfort.

IDEAL STARTING POSITION

The ideal starting position is half prone lying. The client should lie on the right side, with her head turned to the left, left leg and arm slightly bent in front of the body. The right arm is behind the body and the right leg slightly bent. A pillow can be placed underneath the left knee and leg.

METHODS OF RELAXATION: BLOCKING OUT MENTAL IMPULSES

CONTRAST MUSCULAR RELAXATION AND TENSION

In order to know whether muscles are relaxed or tensed they must first be deliberately tensed. Experiencing the sensation of strong muscular contractions is then contrasted with the sensation felt when it is released, which is known as relaxation of the muscle. There are no nerve impulses which produce relaxation, only those which produce a contraction and tension. One method is to contract and relax all the muscle groups consecutively in one session; and another method is to concentrate on one muscle group alone for the whole session before proceeding to another group at the next session.

B.M.—9

BREATHING

The use of deep diaphragmatic breathing, followed by shallower lateral costal and apical breathing is another method by which relaxation is taught.

COLOUR BLACK OR PLEASING OBJECT

This method teaches the client to concentrate solely on emptying the mind and filling it with the colour of black allowing no other penetration of thoughts to enter. Concentration on a pleasant subject, one which fills the mind with warmth, or a special person the client holds dear, the sun, sand drifting through the fingers, the sea, a star, are a few objects which could be suggested and which she must examine, dissect, analyse, criticize, and think about utterly and completely, blocking the way for anything else that might come creeping into her mind. This will lead eventually to her mind being completely blank, first perhaps for only a second or two and then gradually for longer periods of time. At first she may drift into sleep but when the practice period is complete she will be able to use this method, or the other, at any time to empty her mind and relax without sleeping.

COMBINATION

All three methods of relaxing the mind and body can be combined to produce a greater effect, like a doctor's prescription which very often may contain several drugs for their cumulative effect. This is the method, the technique of which will be described in more detail in the following paragraphs. The beauty therapist should practise it herself first so that she is relaxed and can reap the rewards both health- and beauty-wise. She will then be better qualified and able to teach her client how to relax. The same rules apply to her as a client. If at first the therapist does not succeed in relaxing then she should try again and again. When teaching the client to relax, it is important to use a dull, monotonous tone of voice, the speed of which should be slow and consistent.

TECHNIQUE

Feet first. Curl the toes and pull up the ankles as hard as possible. Go on tightening and pulling up. Now let go. Repeat this five times or until the tension can be felt flowing out of the muscles, the foot and ankle becoming heavy and relaxed. Concentrate on the lightening and relaxing, putting all other thoughts out of the mind.

Thigh and seat muscles. Brace the thigh muscles statically pressing the knees back but without movement. Squeeze the seat muscles as hard as possible together, then let go. Repeat even harder and stronger, then gradually let go, feeling the release of tension and muscle tone. Do not allow the mind to wander from tightening and then relaxing.

Hands, wrists, and fingers. Clench the fists very tightly until the fingers dig into the palms of the hands and pull back the wrists as hard as possible. Hold these contractions until it aches, then let go and feel the relief as the aching dies away. Repeat this stronger and stronger about five times more. The rest period between each contraction will become longer as the tension takes longer to ease away after a hard contraction. All sounds around fade and drift away. Just tighten and relax.

Shoulders, upper arms, and back. Press the upper arms into the sides of the body and pull back the shoulders tightly. Hold it and then let go. With each contraction squeeze and tighten a little harder, a little longer, before letting go. This should be done about five times in all. Keep on tightening and letting go, feeling heavier and heavier.

Facial muscles last. Press lips together, screw up the eyes tightly, depress the nose, and clench the teeth, then let go. Again tighten and relax and yet again and again.

The difference between tension and relaxation of muscles groups should now have been learned. The body and mind should now be prepared to float off into sleep.

The whole body. Tighten all the muscle groups of the body and whilst relaxing just concentrate on feeling heavy, limp, and sleepy, shutting out the world completely. Become aware of the comfortable bed and sink into it deeper and deeper. Again, slowly tighten each muscle group and check how tight and tense it is before letting go. As the tension is relaxed, sigh out in relief with nothing at all in the mind but comfort, peace, and physical heaviness. Over and over again. If the emptiness does not blur into a haze and then drift into sleep try the soothing relaxing breathing. Remember there is no hurry; time should be taken the whole way through.

Deep breathing. Begin by taking a deep breath in through the nose allowing the air to fill and expand the chest and push out the abdomen. Slowly sigh out the air through the mouth. Breathe in again feeling heavy and relaxed. Repeat this deep breathing with emphasis on the sighing out. There is no hurry at all between each breath. Each sigh out should be accompanied by allowing the body to sink heavier and heavier like lead into the bed. No thought or sound should distract the mind from this rhythm of deep breathing. Breathe in through the nose even more deeply and sigh out again through the mouth. Gradually change deep breathing into a lighter shallower type by closing the mouth and breathing in and out naturally through the nose. Concentrate on breathing in, and out, in, and out. Push away any thought that creeps into the mind other than the movement of the chest which lifts up, and down, up and down. By now not even the breathing should be apparent and even the gentlest thoughts of regular rhythmic respirations will have become a hypnotic haze and deep sleep should have engulfed the body and the mind. If one small spark of resistance is left allow the mind to become completely absorbed with the colour of black. When a tiny thought wanders into the corner of the mind, black it out, still breathing rhythmically, and relax. Keep bringing the thoughts back to blackness and nothing, slip one second of nothing into the mind and then try another, and yet another. . . .

Having learnt to drift into sleep by one or another of the

methods described above, the therapist should try to practise the relaxation without the sleep. The client should be advised to do the same. This can be done anywhere; there is no need to lie down. She should be encouraged to take time off to relax and leave the rushing, running, and racing for tomorrow.

12. *About Electrical Treatments*

To the professional beauty therapist a fundamental knowledge of electricity is essential. The range and variety of electrical equipment is so vast that it is impossible to keep track of the latest piece, but the basic principles of working remain the same for each type of current used. Galvanic, faradic, sinusoidal, and high-frequency currents are those most commonly utilized for cosmetic purposes, although the direct current is little used today. Together with radiant heat, infra-red, and ultra-violet radiation, they provide some of the many methods of treatment that the therapist will be required to employ during her career. Both in electro-therapy and actino-therapy the highest level of skill, attention, and care in the use of machines is required to produce good results and legitimate effects safely. This basic knowledge of the currents being employed and the effects on the tissues of the body cannot be learned overnight, or with the manufacturer's instructions in one hand and the client in the other. There are several dangers resulting from poor technique, inexperience, and inadequate knowledge which can be fatal and crippling for life. A doctor should always be consulted before electrical treatments are commenced, however well qualified the therapist is.

General Dangers

SHOCKS

The greatest danger when using electrical machines is that of giving an electric shock by earthing as the client becomes part of the circuit. Metal pipes, radiators, wet or stone floors, and metal beds are all conductors to earth if contact is made with a faulty piece of machinery or socket. The more current passing through the client the stronger the shock will be. If the machine is inadequately earthed very severe shocks could occur when treating the limbs in water. Strong currents through the head, neck, or heart, or if the client is totally immersed in water or steam, could be fatal.

To prevent earthing through the client, all apparatus should be properly insulated and each part earthed correctly so that there is no danger of touching a piece of an unearthed 'live' equipment. This is usually guaranteed by the good name of a reliable manufacturer who has to comply to a certain standard. The apparatus should be overhauled regularly by a professional electrical engineer and one who is preferably experienced in the maintenance of medical-electrical and cosmetic equipment. Keep the apparatus away from the client in case of leakage, faulty connections, and wear and tear on insulations. As rubber is a good insulator the therapist should wear rubber-soled shoes for safety, so that she is protected in case of accidents and can safely touch the client in an emergency without herself being earthed. A rubber sheet placed under the linen sheet on the couch, or a rubber mat under the client's feet on the ground is advisable when using electricity, especially with water.

Shocks may also be caused by pure carelessness, not being of the earthing kind at all, but merely an unpleasant and unexpected sensation from the electrical currents. The current sensations should always be explained carefully to the client first and tried out by the therapist on herself in front of the client. If the intensity control switch on the apparatus is not turned down to zero before switching off the equipment after each treatment, a large amount of current may be carelessly passed through the next client when the machine is used again. All apparatus control switches should be turned down to zero or off, before switching on. The selector switch must be carefully checked. Shock-provoking tactics are caused through the current being suddenly increased or decreased due to faulty connections, broken leads, electric power failures, and bad technique. Precautionary measures, in testing the current first to find out if there are any irregularities in the sensation which might give the client a shock, should be taken first before applying it. Increase and decrease the current intensity slowly, especially in water. Contacts on the skin should be firm unless a special effect as in high frequency is required when the glass electrodes should be dry. Special lubricants and contact soaps should be used or talcum powder if a dry surface is required. Broken leads should not be used and the wall socket should always be switched off first before being unplugged.

Do not allow clients to regulate or supervise their own treatments under any circumstances, or come into contact with each other whilst undergoing electrical treatments.

Other untoward effects, such as burns and painful treatments, can be caused through bad technique of application. Faintness can occur due to too much heat or a current on the head or near the heart. The intensity of the treatment may be excessive and duration too long, causing a fall in blood pressure or other signs of stress in the client.

Further General Precautions

1. Care must be taken not to use currents of electricity that would produce haemorrhage, especially after a recent injury to a part, though it is highly unlikely that the client would be at the beauty salon if she had badly injured herself. This principle applies to varicosed and bruised areas.
2. A skin test must always be made before applying electrical currents to make sure that skin sensations are normal. The area being treated is tested for hot and cold, and for sensitivity to a painful stimulus such as a pin prick. This latter can be done by applying the faradaic current to the area.
3. Jewellery should be removed from the part to be treated, especially rings.
4. Skin rash due to sensitivity from currents should be noted and further treatment on this area avoided or delayed. Some skins are more sensitive to certain treatments than others. If there

are any small skin lesions or spots in the area they should be insulated with vaseline before treatment commences.

5. Skin inflammation: treatment should never be given over inflamed areas.
6. Heart: great care should be taken when applying any treatment near the heart.
7. The client must never be permitted to interfere with or touch the equipment.
8. The therapist should be within earshot of the client and be able to see her throughout the treatment, checking at regular intervals that she is all right.

Galvanic Current

PRECAUTIONS FOR THE PREVENTION OF SHOCKS, BURNS AND INJURIES

1. The area must be properly washed, inspected, and prepared before treatment to lower and equalize the resistance of the skin.
2. A skin test for hot and cold should be given prior to treatment and also to test whether the area is anaesthetized. This can be given by using a faradic current or a pin prick. Galvanism should never be given to an anaesthetized area.
3. Cuts or scratches should be insulated with vaseline to prevent current concentration on them.
4. The client should be warm and comfortable.
5. The pads used to cover the electrodes should be made of lint towelling and should be neatly folded, allowing the edges to be even and at least half an inch thick or sixteen lint thicknesses. All the metal must be equally covered before the pads are placed in contact with the client. They should be preferably smaller than the size of the lint pad and made of malleable metal so that they will mould to the shape of the client. The corners should be rounded so that there is no current concentration. The leads and metal clips must also be insulated from the client.

6. The lint should be soaked and wrung out evenly in a one per cent salt solution. (The salt should be allowed to dissolve properly in the hot water.)

7. According to which effect of galvanism is required, other solutions containing drugs can be used and the pads placed accordingly on the part and body.

8. The tingling sensation of galvanism should first be explained to the client before any current is experienced. She must be told most carefully to report if she feels an unevenness of current in the pads, or concentration of heat on one spot, or pain of any description. If this happens, the area should be examined and if one small area is red the treatment should be discontinued as continuation might lead to a serious galvanic burn, deep into the tissues. The amount of current passed through a client very often depends upon the information the client gives, but must not exceed 2 milliamperes per square inch (0·31 mA per square centimetre) of pad under all circumstances. Usually it is much less.

9. Do not allow the client to be misguided into believing that the stronger the current the better the treatment, otherwise a serious burn may occur; therefore do not allow the density to be too high.

10. The current must be given time to adjust to the resistance of the tissues before increasing the intensity.

11. Pressure from bandaging to hold the pad and electrode in place must be even. Protect the bandage from the wet lint pads by rubberized jaconet or rubber, otherwise it may conduct the current. Also protect the linen from becoming wet with a piece of rubber and a towel under the part being treated.

12. Rings and metal in the area must be removed.

13. The client must not touch any electrodes.

14. Rest the client's feet on a rubber mat if she is in a sitting position.

15. A different area should be treated each day.

16. Depending upon which effect is required, so the length of duration of treatment will vary.

17. On completion of treatment the current must be turned off slowly.
18. The skin should be washed to remove acids and well dried.
19. The exact details and reaction of the treatments must be precisely recorded. This includes the size of pads, area of treatment, solution used, current intensity, and duration of treatment.

Faradism and Sinusoidal Currents

PRECAUTIONARY MEASURES FOR THE COMFORT OF THE CLIENT

1. Burns cannot occur with these currents but if technique is poor they can be painful and uncomfortable. If the client is totally immersed in a bath the current should be earth free. These currents must be surged to make the muscles contract and relax.
2. The beauty therapist should test the current on herself first before applying it to the client.
3. The sensations of the current must be carefully explained before use on the client.
4. The client must be comfortable and warm, and all water used in treatments should be a hot one per cent salt solution.
5. Electrodes and pads can be conveniently fixed to the area with rubber straps. The pads must be thoroughly soaked in the water and the area moistened if necessary.
6. Smooth surging of these currents with a period of relaxation between the contractions is vital for comfort. A long sustained contraction is tiring and fatiguing.
7. For greater skin stimulation the sinusoidal current is preferable. Muscle contractions are obtained with the surged faradaic current. Uninterrupted stimulation causes a temporary deadening effect.
8. When a group of muscles is stimulated the indifferent pad should be placed on either the nerve trunk or a convenient area of skin nearby or the origin of the muscles. The active

electrode should be placed over the motor point of the muscles or over their insertion.

9. The duration of treatment should be rapidly progressed to a maximum of twenty minutes. Uninterrupted stimulation on a small area should last for only about five minutes. If the labile and bath methods are used, ten to twenty minutes, depending on the current density, is sufficient.

10. The current density depends upon the client's tolerance of it, but for muscle toning with surged faradaism a good strong contraction is required, to be of any value.

11. The current intensity should be turned on and off slowly at the commencement and end of treatment when all parts should be well dried and powdered.

12. The client should be allowed to rest if she wishes to do so but this is not essential.

13. The treatment should be recorded accurately.

Infra-red and Radiant Heat Radiation

DANGERS

1. Burns may occur if the client is too close to the lamp, if she touches it, or if the intensity is too high.

2. Some clients are misguided enough to think that the lamp has to burn and feel very hot for maximum benefit.

3. If the circulation is poor a burn may occur because the area heats up but the blood does not circulate and disperse the heat.

4. Skin should be washed clean and free from oils, unguents, and linaments which could cause burning and painful blisters.

5. The muslin can catch fire if too near the lamp.

6. Earth shocks may occur if insulation is faulty and the client touches the lamp.

7. Dizziness and faintness can be caused, due to a fall in blood pressure produced by excess heat.

8. Headaches and nausea may occur with radiant heat bath treatments, especially if the client does not sweat. Cold compresses can be placed on the client's head.

9. Extra water should be drunk unless a weight loss is desired.
10. General irradiation in a heat bath is not given during very hot weather and the time for local irradiation is reduced to a minimum. This depends upon the size of the lamp but should be measured from its element. Usually eighteen to twenty-four inches (46 to 60 cm) is the correct distance away from the skin to produce a slight erythema and gentle warmth of the tissues in ten minutes. Many lamps carry the manufacturer's instructions which should be tested before use. Every client will have a different reaction so no rule is hard and fast. After the first ten minutes the heat can be increased if required by turning up the intensity control or moving the lamp closer. Up to half an hour's exposure is sufficient.
11. The lamp must never be placed directly over the client as this can be dangerous and cause a burn if any part of it were to fall on her.

RADIANT HEAT RADIATION (R.H.)

This form of heating feels milder than I.R.R., but it can still burn the skin and produce unpleasant scorch marks which could take several weeks to disappear.

PRECAUTIONS

1. Test the skin sensation for hot and cold.
2. Cover sensitive areas with a muslin cloth to prevent scorching from the bulb.
3. Place a blanket over both ends of the bath type of radiant heat to allow a more even heating of the skin. If the ends of a bath are left open to allow air to flow through it, scorching is more likely.
4. The lamp should be placed at a distance of eighteen to twenty-four inches (46 to 60 cm) away.
5. Position the lamp parallel to the part.
6. Turn on the lamp before use to allow it to warm up, particularly with the bath cabinet.

7. Between twenty and thirty minutes is a sufficient length of time for exposure.
8. Check temperature of client before and during treatment in a bath. Do not allow a rise of more than one or two degrees Fahrenheit (half to one degree Centigrade).
9. Do not leave the client alone for too long; keep checking at regular intervals to see that she is feeling all right.
10. Allow the client to rest and cool down after treatment.
11. A cool shower or bath to wash away sweat and reduce the body temperature to normal should be available before the client leaves the salon.

Ultra-violet Light (U.V.L.)

There is no immediate effect of pinking to be seen on the skin on treatment with ultra-violet rays. This pinking is called an erythema and it appears four to six hours after irradiation. There are four degrees of erythema but only the first two are usually used in beauty therapy. A first degree erythema or E_1 fades after twenty-four hours and there is no skin peeling. A second degree erythema or E_2 is a stronger pinking or reddening of the skin and fades after two or three days followed by fine peeling. A sub-erythemal dose is one which does not produce any visible reaction in the skin at all.

DANGERS

1. Severe burns can arise from careless use.
2. Blindness can occur if the eyes are not protected with special goggles.
3. U.V.L. can be dangerous if given to people with heart disease, nephritis, arterio-sclerosis, Addison's disease, or exophthalmic goitre.
4. Irritation of the skin can occur.
5. Other eruptions of the skin can occur.
6. Headaches, vomiting, increased irritability, sleeplessness, or other symptoms can develop through exposure to U.V.L.

7. If a client is taking certain drugs U.V.L. could be dangerous.
8. Earthing could occur if the client touched the burner.
9. Chills can occur if the room is cold or draughty.

PRECAUTIONS

1. Each time the lamp is used the number of minutes should be recorded in a special book, as the rays become weaker with use, and longer exposures are required with an old lamp than with a new.

2. The erythema reaction should be tested on the client first to ascertain the dosage. If the stated dosage produces an E_1 in one minute, the test doses would be given for half, one, and one and a half minutes. The client would be asked to note very carefully how long afterwards the erythema showed up and for how long it lasted.

3. The distance from the lamp varies with each lamp and usually the manufacturer encloses a leaflet of instructions which should be followed precisely and tested. If these are not available, the lamp should be tested at one, two, and three feet away (or at 33 cm, 67 cm, and 1 metre away) for the first degree erythema dose.

4. It is important to place the lamp parallel to the surface being treated so that the rays strike the skin at right angles and maximum absorption is obtained into the skin.

5. The temperature of the skin can alter the effect of the treatment for it is more sensitive to U.V.L. when warm than when cold.

6. Infra-red and radiant heat rays can increase sensitivity if given before ultra-violet radiation but diminish the effect if given afterwards. In this last way they can be used as an antidote to an overdose.

7. Skin colourings differ in reaction to U.V.L. Fair skins are usually more sensitive than dark skins. Certain areas of the body are more sensitive than others, therefore the erythema dose may vary from one part to another.

8. The dose is increased by lengthening the time of exposure.

To maintain a first degree erythema, up to four minutes can be added by increasing the time by twenty-five per cent each session. After that only one minute at a time should be added for a maximum of twenty minutes. Three times a week is desirable but daily doses can be given. If the client misses her treatment the dosage should not be increased up to ten days, half the dosage up to fourteen days and the original dose if longer.

9. If an overdose occurs, infra-red rays should be applied to the area immediately. This will have the effect of producing an I.R.R. erythema which will reduce the intensity of the ultraviolet rays. Cold cream can be applied to the part, and later, if necessary, calamine lotion is cooling and soothing.

10. Care must be taken to expose the same area of skin for each treatment.

11. If the lamp goes out the client must not touch the lamp.

12. The beauty therapist must wear special goggles all the time.

13. Good ventilation is necessary to keep the room free from fumes.

14. The room must be warm.

15. Keep the lamp low down and face down to the floor before use.

16. Strike the lamp five minutes before irradiation and leave on till all treatments are completed.

17. The parts around the area to be irradiated must be protected and until the lamp is correctly positioned the part to be treated must be covered.

18. The therapist must not touch the filament or burner of the lamp.

19. The lamp must never be positioned directly over the client.

High Frequency

PRECAUTIONS

1. Explanation of the sparking effect and a demonstration should be given first on the beauty therapist before use on the client.

2. The area to be treated must be thoroughly dry.

3. The electrode should be applied to the skin before turning on the current as this avoids frightening the client.
4. For a soothing treatment firm contact with the skin must be maintained to prevent sparking.
5. For stimulation the electrode should only be in light contact with the skin allowing the small sparks to produce a bright erythema effect. If strong stimulation is required the electrode should be lifted further away from the skin, but in these cases a rash may be produced.
6. The skin must be free of any lotions or preparations containing sulphur or alcohol.
7. Do not sit the client near metal pipes or allow jewellery near the area being treated. A wooden chair should be used and she should be comfortable and warm.
8. After use the glass electrodes should be cleaned and sterilized; care must be taken to dry the electrodes before use again.

Some Conditions for Treatments

It is not within the province of the beauty therapist to treat medical conditions. However, she will find that there are many clients who, whilst having massage, electrical, or other cosmetic treatments, will be inclined to mention a pain in the back, a headache, or a gammy knee. These clients should be referred back to their doctor for such conditions, who may then give permission for the beauty therapist to apply heat, or modify the massage to fit the case, and perhaps relieve discomfort in suitable cases. The following conditions are those most widely prevalent. They would only be treated if present to a lesser degree, and not in the acute stages, but the doctor would decide whether they were suitable cases for beauty therapy.

ARTHRITIS, RHEUMATISM, AND OTHER CONDITIONS

These are terms used to denote a pain, ache, or stiffness in joints, muscles, and bones. In actual fact they can be likened to the surname of a large family of individual conditions which produce these symptoms.

B.M.—9*

RHEUMATOID ARTHRITIS

Rheumatoid arthritis is a condition of the joints where the synovial membranes are affected, generally in the smaller joints of the body. It is apparently more common in females than in males, and the onset is between twenty and forty years of age. The fingers and toes can take on a spindle shaped appearance because the joints swell and thicken, and the muscles above and below the joints dwindle and atrophy, and they can become quite deformed in advanced cases. In the acute stages the joints are very hot and shiny and must be left alone.

Cause: thought to be a focal infection such as tonsillitis or excessive wear and tear if only one joint is affected. Generally the cause is unknown.

Treatment: Mild radiant heat, passive exercises, active exercises. Massage to the wasted muscles but avoided at all times on the affected joints. Wax baths can be given to the hands and feet and this is a most popular form of treatment.

OSTEO-ARTHRITIS

Osteo-arthritis is less crippling than the bad cases of rheumatoid arthritis. It affects large weight-bearing joints mainly and is a disease of middle and later life. The cartilage of the joints wears away exposing the bone which hardens. The synovial membrane may calcify and chip off into the joint, limiting movement. Osteo-arthritis of the knees is most commonly seen in large obese women. The therapist may find the joints creak on movement, and patella movements are restricted.

Cause is thought to be poor postural habits, metabolic changes, occupational stress, and strain on joints.

Treatment: Heat treatment such as infra-red radiation. Vigorous joint massage, mobility and strengthening exercises.

FIBROSITIS

Fibrositis is a painful rheumatic condition affecting all ages, more common in men than women. It takes the form of deep-seated tender nodules which at times can be excessively painful and quite incapacitating. Sometimes during a massage the therapist may discover a tender spot particularly in the back muscles. The therapist should be able to feel these areas; the client certainly will.

Cause: The schools of thought about fibrositis vary. Some say the nodules are fatty globules caught up in the muscle fibres; others say that they are areas of tension in the muscle fibres. Muscle strain, a focal infection such as a bad tooth, or exposure to cold, wet, and damp conditions are all contributory factors.

Treatment: Heat treatment such as I.R.R. or R.H. or other available heat. Massage with deep frictions and effleurage. Exercises.

TENOSYNOVITIS

Tenosynovitis is the inflammation of the synovial sheath and membrane of the tendon of a muscle. Most commonly found in the tendons of the wrist or ankle. In the acute stage there is much swelling, pain, and even crepitus (creaking) on movement. The doctor will probably order rest and apply a strapping to the part. It should be left completely alone until it has subsided.

Cause: Unknown—probably overuse or strain of the muscle.

Treatment: Gentle heat. Faradic hand bath may be given. Gentle finger kneadings.

TENNIS ELBOW

Tennis elbow is a fibrositic condition round the elbow. Occurs not only in tennis players, but in many housewives who carry heavy shopping bags or who suddenly attempt to paint the house. The area is a tender spot found in the common extensor tendon of the forearm, around the head of the radius, and around the back of the lateral condyle of the humerus. Sometimes it is the supinator muscle of the forearm.

Cause: muscle strain is most commonly attributed to the cause.

Treatment: Heat treatment, infra-red, anodal galvanism. Massage with deep transverse frictions across the belly of the muscle into the affected area. Eccentric muscle work exercises for the extensors of the forearm.

FROZEN SHOULDER

Frozen shoulder is a 'rheumaticky' condition around the shoulder area resulting in pain and stiffness on abduction of the arm. It can vary from complete loss of movement to a mild twinge in the shoulder region.

Cause: fibrositis in the supra-spinatus tendon.

Treatment: Heat treatment. Massage and exercises for the shoulder girdle muscles.

LUMBAGO

Lumbago can describe the form of a dull heavy intense low back-ache in the lumbar vertebrae region. It may hinder movement.

Cause can be due to bad posture, extra physical exertion, lifting heavy weights, nursing mothers, bad stance in massage practice (occupational causes).

Treatment: Deep massage over origin of latissimus dorsi, the erector spinae muscles, and the lumbar region. Ironing, finger kneadings, and effleurage. Heat treatment. Back extension exercises.

SCIATICA

Sciatica can denote pain in the lumbar region, sacral region down the back of the leg from the buttocks, sacro-iliac and hip joint.

Cause is pressure on the sciatic nerve (which travels from the lower lumbar vertebrae down into the back of the thigh) due to wear and tear of lumbar joints and bones, bad posture, also tumours or tuberculosis both of which would not be treated.

Treatment: Heat treatment. Massage, ironing, finger kneadings, and frictions around the lumbar, sacro-iliac joints, and sacrum. Exercises correcting pelvic tilt and posture and back extension exercises.

SLIPPED DISK

Slipped disk is the forward protrusion of the cartilage found between the bodies of the vertebrae. One or more lesions may occur and they are most commonly found in the cervical and lumbar regions of the spine. Great care is necessary at all times if a client is thought to be suffering from a slipped disk. Flexion of the spine should be avoided and she should be taught how to bend from the knees and hips keeping the back rigid and straight. She should have a doctor's note authorizing all cosmetic treatment to the body.

Cause: lifting heavy weights, muscle weakness, strain on the joints, wear and tear of the joints.

Treatment: Heat treatment. Back extension exercises with particular emphasis on strengthening exercises.

FLAT FEET

This condition can be taken to mean one of several in the feet. It can mean an outward turning of the feet; it can mean a foot which is banged down heavily with each footstep like a piece of wood; or it can mean a complete or partial collapse of one or both arches of the feet. The most important aim when treating any variety of flat foot is to keep it mobile and functional.

Cause. Various causes are attributed to flat feet conditions. They can be due to hereditary factors, strain, overweight, injury, ill-fitting shoes, or weak muscles, to mention but a few.

Treatment: Deep massage to the sole of the foot and to the tibialis anterior muscle which is one of the chief supports of the medial arch of the foot. Faradic foot baths to all the arches of the feet. Active exercises, both mobility and strengthening exercises should be given.

SKIN CONDITIONS

ACNE VULGARIS

This is an unsightly condition occurring mainly in adolescence. It tends to clear up by itself after the age of twenty-one. The regions mainly affected are the face, between the scapulae, over the sternal region and possibly the neck. It is characterized by comedos (blackheads) and raised pustules on the skin which is usually greasy.

Cause: said to be a maladjustment of the sebaceous glands at this stage of life.

Treatment: Ultra-violet light (an E_2) is given to the areas, care being taken to clean and wipe off any grease first which would filter off some of the rays preventing them from penetrating. The face should be treated in sections so that the lamp can be accurately positioned parallel to its shape. All areas not being treated must be covered and an accurate skin test should be performed before treatment commences. The eyes should be protected with vaseline and covered with cotton wool.

BLACKHEADS

Blackheads can be expressed with a sterile blackhead expressor.

BOILS AND CARBUNCLES

A boil is an inflamed and septic area of the subcutaneous tissues and skin containing pus and a hard core. A carbuncle can be several boils confined to one local area, or an exceptionally large local inflammation containing pus and a core.

Cause: various causes such as lowered resistance to infection, or greasy dirty clogged infected pores.

Treatment: After the inflammation has subsided and the infection cleared a general tonic course of sunlight treatment could be given. This would be a first degree erythema dose of three treatments weekly for six to eight weeks' duration.

PSORIASIS

This condition is a non-infectious skin condition which can be confined to one small area or in sporadic patches all over the body. It is characterized by round red raised dry patches covered with silvery scales. It seems to appear on the extensor surfaces of the body, but can occur either surface. For instance, it appears on the back of the arms, on the front of the legs, and on the back of the trunk. The scalp can also be affected at the roots of the hair.

Cause seems to be constitutional and can appear in early childhood, then disappear, and reappear again at any crisis in life.

Treatment: Oil massage has been found to be helpful. General sunlight treatment may help.

Pine tar baths may help, followed by a brisk towelling down and an oil massage to loosen the dry scales.

High frequency can be given to the scalp, the showers of sparks help to increase the circulation.

N.B. By improving the condition of the skin, scaling may be prevented and also skin infections, common in this condition.

ALOPECIA

There are two types of alopecia:

1. *Alopecia areata* affects localized areas of the scalp and is characterized by small round areas of baldness mainly on occipital region of the cranium, but it can spread to the parietal bones. The patches may be up to an inch across single or in groups.
2. *Alopecia totalis* affects the whole scalp and eyebrows. ('Senile' alopecia affecting men, rarely women, begins in the thirties or perhaps earlier, and is a condition in which the hair begins to recede from the temples, or in the crown of the head spreading outwards).

Course. When the hair begins to grow again it is at first white or blonde and very fair. After a length of time the downy hair is replaced by normal hair, but it is white and only after many months does the hair become pigmented again.

Cause is thought to be partly psychological, but unknown.

Treatment: This is usually given to relieve nervous tension and can take several forms, which will help to tone up the general health of the body. A course of massage and exercises could be given. The massage would be soothing and relaxing following the exercises, either a general course of sunlight treatment or a localized treatment of the area.

Localized treatment would try to improve the circulation of the scalp by using high frequency or a second degree dose of sunlight. It is passed over the area where the hair is expected to grow and is used every other day. Ultra-violet radiation, giving an E_2 in cases of alopecia totalis, would involve sectioning the scalp into four areas, that is the two sides, top, and back. The face and ears should be covered and the client could hold a towel over them. The two sides would be treated first and then the top and back of the head would be treated four days after when the first E_2 had died down. The dosage may become longer as it is increased each time; however, if it becomes too long, then high frequency may be used instead every other day. A whole head should take about twenty minutes to treat.

IMPETIGO

This is a highly infectious acute skin infection which should on no account be treated but referred immediately to the doctor. Small vesicles appear on the surface of the skin which are filled with a clear fluid thick with bacteria. It appears on the face and ears and is carried anywhere on the body by scratching. Wherever the fluid is spread impetigo will spring up. It is most commonly found in dirty people and spread around communities if it is not spotted and treated medically.

NAEVUS

This condition is a small area of dilated blood vessels to be found on the skin. Sometimes they form a purple area on the skin and are known as a port wine stain or birthmark. The port wine stain is very difficult to cure. With strong local doses of ultra-violet light they may fade but are rarely cured. The most superficial naevus may be treated by a galvanic current or high frequency in an attempt to try and disperse the fine vein-like threads of blood. It is doubtful that these conditions can be influenced at all by treatment, and many beauty therapists leave them alone.

SUPERFLUOUS HAIRS

This condition is thought to be due to the incorrect balance of hormones. Sometimes the cause is attributed to heredity but generally thought to be glandular. It can occur in young people who should be advised by their doctor, but more frequently, when the hormone balance is disturbed, it is during the menopause. It is a condition which requires a specially trained therapist with great tact and understanding.

Treatment: There are varying forms of treatment which range from waxing to using depilatories. Electrolysis is frequently and most satisfactorily used on the face but unless it is expertly administered the hair will grow again. The needle must be inserted down the hair follicle in order to destroy the root of the hair, and care must be taken to use the right polarity to destroy the hair, otherwise a black charring scar will result.

WARTS

Before attempting treatment of warts the doctor should be consulted. If treatment is recommended electrolysis, magnesium drugs, or a third degree erythema dose of sunlight can be effective. High frequency is a popular method of treating warts.

DEBILITY

A general tired run-down condition of the client which can be due to several factors. It could be anaemia, overwork, aftermath of illness, constant coughs and colds, poor appetite. The client would be advised to seek the advice of the doctor before commencing treatment to ascertain the cause.

Treatment: General light massage and exercises.

A course of sunlight treatment consisting of a sub-erythema dose, gradually increasing to a first degree dose of ultra-violet light, could prove to be most beneficial.

Care of Equipment

A bad workman blames his tools and no matter how superb the technique of treatment may be, if the equipment is neglected the final performance can only be at a sub-standard level. Great personal pride in handling and looking after equipment and materials lies in conjunction with good workmanship. To see a well-cared-for department or salon is both encouraging and reassuring to the client. A neat shining orderly salon reflects the pride and interest taken by those who work in it. One which is higgledy-piggledy is not conducive to a peaceful and calm atmosphere, neither does it create a favourable impression.

Hints on Orderliness

1. *Tidiness* of the couch and linen is important. When folding sheets, blankets, and towels, make a point of folding the edges neatly inside. Turn the pillow case opening away from the door. Tuck the corners of the sheets into the couch like an envelope corner. Place used towels neatly into a laundry bin. Place a bowl on the trolley for cotton wool or used tissues.

2. *Machinery* should be kept in one place, regularly dusted, the shining reflectors and chrome polished, enamel carefully washed. When not in use they should be covered with dust

sheets which in turn must be regularly washed. The face of the heat and sunlight lamps should be turned to the floor and lowered down as far as possible, the wires wrapped carefully round the hooks provided on the machines. All switches and controls should be at zero and the plugs removed from the sockets which should be switched off. Any damaged or broken equipment should be repaired immediately and not left until required for treatment again. Leads should be neatly hung up or separated in a box; rubber straps and bandages likewise. Most manufacturers send cleaning instructions for their equipment.

3. *The store cupboards* must be thoroughly cleaned once a week and tidied every day.
4. *The floors* should be cleaned every day.
5. *Electrodes* must be stored dry and flat, especially if metal.
6. *Lint pads* washed out and renewed when necessary.
7. *Sometimes sterilization* of equipment is essential, especially needles which are used for electrolysis.
8. *Small jars* and bottles should be kept topped up from larger containers and drips wiped away.
9. *A waste bin* should be lined with paper, unless disposal bags are used.
10. *All linen* and gown frequently changed and washed.

Help the Client

1. The therapist can help the client to sit up by hooking her near arm through the client's, with the other arm firmly encircled round the client's back.
2. Stand near the client when she stands up, from lying or sitting, or after having had a course of heat treatment, whether in a steam bath or dry heat, in case of dizziness.
3. Pick up the client's shoes for her, and hand her a gown or her clothes.
4. Call her by her name.
5. Show her to the couch and show her right to the door when she leaves.

6. Present the account simply after each treatment, or at the end of the course of treatment.
7. Do not rush the client.
8. Be a good listener by being genuinely interested in the client's welfare.

13. *New Techniques*

Aromatherapy

The word 'aromatherapy' is derived from 'aroma' meaning odour of oil and 'therapy' meaning the art of applying.

EFFECTS AND USES

The more concentrated the oil the more effective it is, and therefore the more beneficial aromatherapy is to mind and body. It is claimed that aromatherapy improves health through the use of certain essential oils and gives the client a sense of well-being.

With the use of certain oils on some problem skins, aromatherapy can improve the texture and revitalize the skin giving it a feeling of beauty.

Certain aromatic colours can relax a nervous or tense client and this can be very beneficial. It is also claimed that some aromatic scents, if used on the correct problem and client, can stimulate the mind to make the client feel more alert and bright.

PROCEDURE

The order and method of work and the preparation and procedure should be the same as described in Chapter 5. (The actual massage movements are explained below.) A client record card should be filled in as normal with a note of which oil has been chosen and why. The therapist should use her skill in choosing a correct aromatic oil after talking to the client gently and assessing the problem for which the client most needs help. It may be that the client has certain skin problems on her body or face which she feels she would like to improve or perhaps she cannot sleep at night and has a need for relaxation. It is then up to the therapist to determine the real reason for the treatment so that the correct essential oil can be chosen.

THE ART OF APPLYING AND TECHNIQUES OF AROMATHERAPY

There are forty-three pressure points on the anterior part of the body which is where the therapist begins her massage. The client must be in a comfortable position and the room must be very warm so that the client will not feel cold when the towel is removed from the area on which the therapist is working.

The therapist sits at the end of the bed with the chosen essential oil in bowls at either side of the client's feet. Starting at the toes, the therapist works her way up the body applying the oil to each pressure point with a certain amount of pressure in her middle fingers. Once she has applied all the oil to the pressure points on the body she begins again using only effleurage movements, working her way from the points at the feet to the arms from one pressure point to the next, massaging slowly and rhythmically until she feels the client relax.

When the massage to the front of the body has been completed the client should turn over and the same procedure should be followed. There are ninety pressure points on the posterior side of the body, most of which are on the back. Care and time must be taken on the client's back for if she has not yet relaxed this is her last chance and the treatment will have been a success.

If the client is being given an aromatic facial, then again the same procedure must be followed. The pressure points of the face must be learnt thoroughly by the therapist before she attempts this type of treatment.

AROMATIC OILS – THEIR PROPERTIES AND USES

Rose: antibacteriological, mature dry sensitive skins, soothing effect, headaches, anti-depressant.

Sage: stimulant, astringent, fluid retention, stiff necks, rheumatism, fibrositis, all aches and pains.

Tangerine: revitalizing, tonic for children and young people, pale complexions, improves circulation.

Thyme: strong general stimulant, dermatitis, boils.

Eucalyptus: chest rubs, nasal bronchitis, muscular pains, insect bite wounds.

Juniper: antiseptic, astringent, acne, stimulates circulation and blood purifier, dermatitis, psoriasis, oily skins, cleansing, toning.

Lemon grass: astringent, tired legs, venous conditions, strong antibacterial effects.

Marjoram: nervous tension, good bath oil, warming, calming, relieving pain, rheumatics, sprains, stress, general body massage.

Neroli: non-irritant, eau de cologne, sedative anti-depressant, calms and slows down the mind, all skin types, redness, dryness, broken capillaries, improves skin elasticity, insomnia.

Peppermint: reduces inflamation, decongestion, cooling effects, burns, respiratory problems.

Sandalwood: antiseptic, mild astringent, insomnia, nervous tension, dry skins, sedating purposes, high colour and broken capillaries.

Patchouli: anxiety, depression, skin care, wounds, bactericidal action, aphrodisiac, stimulating in small doses, effect of sedation depending on individual, promotes formation of scar tissue.

FACIAL TREATMENTS

Geranium: for pale complexions.

Sandalwood: for broken capillaries, acneic skins, softening effect.

Lavender: soothes irritation, gives a feeling of freshness.

Basil: antispasmodic, antiseptic, tonic effect, herpes.

Bergamots: antiseptic, anxiety.

Benzoin: for redness, irritation, itching, cracked dry skin, relaxing effect, uplifting.

Camomile: mother herb, burns, boils, dermatitis, acne, allergies, all skin types.

Rosemary: for migraine, rheumatism, muscular pain, dehydrating oil, fluid retention, facial, puffy eyes.

Lavender: for nervous tension, relaxing, uplifting, sensitive acneic skins, antiseptic diuretic properties, wounds, burns, bites, soothing effect on eczema, psoriasis, boils, acne, dermatitis, invigorates body and mind, skin rejuvenation.

Ylang-ylang: for depression, anxiety, nervous tension, oily skins, aphrodisiac, antiseptic, pale complexions, effect of pushing out impurities.

Jasmine mix: for dry sensitive skins, dermatitis, skin elasticity, nervous system, to relieve anxiety and depression.

Gyratory Massage

A gyratory massage machine is used for general body work and is normally floor-standing, with the weight of the motor supported by the main shaft or pedestal of the apparatus.

Sometimes gyratory massage is used simply to complement manual massage but mainly it is an adequate treatment for the removal of cellulite while a client is trying to lose weight.

Gyratory vibrators operate in a vertical and horizontal plane and the therapist can create a circular movement while the massager vibrates up and down.

There are three different types of heads which can be attached to the massager and each one has different effects.

1. *The sponge head*: this must always be used first and has the same effect as effleurage.
2. *The hard rubber ball head*: the same effect as petrissage.
3. *The spiky three-pin heads*: these have the same effect as tapotement.

The feeling and effects of these applicators are totally different from those of manual massage. It is a far deeper massage and breaks down cellulite to the extent of grinding it to the bone on excessively large clients where manual massage would have no effect whatsoever.

Contra-indications
1. Varicose veins.
2. Identified lumps, skin tags, hairy moles.

3. Thrombosis.
4. Pregnancy or during menstruation on abdomen.
5. Very thin or elderly clients.
6. Slipped discs on the back area.
7. Extremely sensitive skins.
8. Excessive hair (usually on men's legs as the pin heads could become caught on the hair and cause extreme discomfort).

EFFECTS

1. Figure improvement, breakdown of cellulite.
2. Increases the blood circulation.
3. Improves the muscular system.
4. Relaxing, especially on large clients.
5. Muscular pain relieved due to the relaxation of tense muscle fibres.
6. Improves skin tone.

METHOD

The client must be prepared in the same way as for body massage and the contra-indications must be carefully checked before commencing the treatment.

Once the therapist has decided which area of the client is to be treated, the gyratory massage talcum powder is spread on the area. This allows the applicator to be massaged over the skin without it dragging and causing discomfort.

The therapist must always begin with the soft foam head for effleurage which prepares the client's skin for a deeper massage. The treatment is applied with long sweeping strokes in an upward direction, always towards the heart. The movements will follow the natural contours of the body and enough pressure must be applied so that it does not cause unnecessary irritation.

The gyratory massage machine is a heavy piece of equipment but with practice and strength in the arms and wrists it becomes an enjoyable and skilful treatment for the therapist.

Depending on the intensity of the problem, the time taken with various applicators will vary. At the end of the treatment the sponge head must always be used as a calming and soothing end to the treatment.

ADVANTAGES OF GYRATORY MASSAGE

1. Adds variety to body treatments.
2. Helps the breakdown of fatty deposits.
3. Less energy-consuming for the therapist.
4. Less personal, so that it can be used for treatment on men.

LOOKING AFTER THE GYRATORY MASSAGER

Gyratory massagers can be very expensive so adequate attention must be paid to this piece of equipment.

1. Regular servicing.
2. Correct use.
3. Correct cleaning and sterilizing of the heads when necessary. A number of each head should be purchased.
4. The heads should only be used with talc and on a clean skin.
5. Never use on oil and make sure that the skin is free from oil if the treatment follows a body massage.
6. Always wash the applicators after use with a mild detergent and allow to dry thoroughly.
7. Dust the dry sterilized sponge with a thin layer of talc before putting it away to keep it in good condition.
8. If the sponge begins to break away from the rubber an apropriate adhesive should be used to bond the two together again.

Index

Abdomen, 40
    distension, 27
    exercises, 225–6, 230–1
    massage, 27, 58, 73–9
Abdominal muscles, 215–19
Abdominal organs, 24
    effect of massage, 32, 35, 36, 49
    kneading, 25
Abdominal wall
    massage technique, 75, 78
    muscles, 167–8
Abduction, 116
Abductor digiti minimi, 157
Abductor hallucis, 157
Abductor pollicis longus, 145
Accounts, 17
Acetabulum, 99
Achilles tendon, 68, 158
Acne vulgaris, 264
Acromio–clavicular joint, 119
Acromion process, 94
Adduction, 116
Adductor brevis, 152
Adductor hallucis obliquis, 157
Adductor hallucis traversus, 157
Adductor longus, 152
Adductor magnus, 152
Adductor muscles, 66
Adhesions, 31, 45, 46
Adipose tissue, see Fatty tissue
Alopecia, 265–6
Anatomical position, 90–1
Anconens, 144
Ankle joints, 93, 102, 103, 126
    exercises, 227–8, 233
    massage technique, 68
    passive movements, 178

Ankle joints—*continued*
    remedying stiffness, 86
Aponeurosis, 136
Appointments, 11, 52
Armpit, see Axilla
Arms, 92, 93
    bones, 94–8
    exercises, 222–3, 228
    forearm, 26, 93
    joints, 119–24
    massage, 57, 61–4
    muscles, 140–5
    passive movements, 175–7
Aromatherapy, 271
Arterio-sclerosis, 40
Arteries, 46
Arthritis, 31, 40
Articular disks, 114
Articularis genu, 151
Asymmetrical exercises, 195
Auricularis, 170
Axilla, 21, 61, 70, 73, 166
Axillary glands, 60

Back
    clapping, 33
    effect of massage, 31, 49
    exercises, 208–9, 224, 229
    flat, 213
    ironing, 28
    massage, 58, 68–72
    muscles, 27, 158–63
Back bone, see Vertebral column
Balance exercises, 195
Beating, 19, 34–5, 43, 72
Beauty salons
    aids to relaxation, 38

Beauty salons—*continued*
  atmosphere, 16
  decor, 16
  orderliness, 268-9
Beauty therapists
  appearance, 11-12, 15, 53
  essential qualities, 9-13
  full-time courses, 8
  relationship to clients, 10-11
  relationship to medical staff, 12-13,
    17
Bedside manner, 9
Biceps, 61, 62, 140, 153
Birch twigs, 3
Blackheads, 264
Blankets, 15, 20, 52
Blood flow, 20
  effect of massage, 30, 33, 46
  See also Circulation
Blood pressure, 40
Blood supply to muscles, 136
Blood vessels in joints, 115
Boils, 264
Bones, 88-110
  classification, 89-90
  effect of exercise, 183
  effect of massage, 45-6
  function, 89
  growth, 45
  marrow, 88-9
  structure, 88
  terminology of features, 90
  types, 88
Brachialis, 140
Brachioradialis, 144
Breast bone, *see* Sternum
Breathing, 234-40
  as aid to relaxation, 244
  exercises, 184, 193, 235-40
  mechanics, 234-5
  relaxed, 238
  types, 236-7, 238
Bronchioles, 47

Buccinator, 170
Bursae, 114
Business organization, 16-18
Bust exercises, 225, 230
Buttocks
  exercises, 226, 231-2
  massage, 59, 72
  muscles, 147, 148

Calcaneum, 103
Calcium, 88, 89
Calf muscles, 67
Capsules (joints), 113
Carbuncles, 264
Carpo-metacarpal joints, 123
Carpus, 97
Cartilage, 88
Centre of gravity, 189-90, 194
Chartered Society of Massage and
    Medical Gymnastics, 7
Chartered Society of Physiotherapy, 7
Chest, 224-5, 230
  massage, 33, 57, 72
  muscles, 163, 165-6
Chin, 110
Circulation, 45
  aided by passive movements, 174
  effect of exercise, 183-4
  effect of massage, 21, 29, 33, 46
  indications of poor circulation, 23
  See also Blood flow
Circumduction, 117-18
City and Guilds of London Institute,
    7-8
Clapping, 19, 33, 43, 66
Clavicle, 21, 91, 94-5
Clients
  help from therapist, 269-70
  position on couch, 53-4
  reception, 53
  relationship to beauty therapist,
    10-11
Coccyx, 105, 106

Collar bone, *see* Clavicle
Colon, 49, 50, 77
Compressor naris, 170
Condyles, 67
Constipation, 27, 34
Contra-indications for massage, 53
Conversation, 13
Cooling, 23
Co-ordination exercises, 195
Coraco-brachialis, 139
Coracoid process, 94
Coronoid fossa, 96
Coronoid process, 96
Corrugator, 170
Cosmetics, 6
Couch, 15, 43, 53-4
Creams, 1, 5-6, 41
Cuboid bone, 103, 104
Cuneiform bones, 103, 104
Cutaneous nerves, 23, 24

Debility, 268
Definitions
    anatomical, 91
    of bone features, 90
Deltoid muscle, 29, 60, 61, 62, 138
Deodorants, 5, 12
Depression (joint movement), 117
Depressor labii inferioris, 170
Depressor septi, 170
Depth of manipulation, 43
Diabetes, 50
Diaphragm, 163-4
Diarrhoea, 40
Digestion, 27, 32, 34, 50, 74, 184
Digital tapotement, *see* Hacking
Dilator naris, 170

Earthing, 248-9
Eau de cologne, 41, 43
Effleurage, 6, 19-22, 31, 36-7, 45-6,
    60, 61, 63, 65-9, 72-3
Elbow joints, 62-3, 85, 93, 120, 175-6
Electric shocks, 248-50

Electrical equipment, 16, 19, 268
Electrical treatments, 248-70
    contra-indications, 250-1
    Faradism, 253-4
    galvanic current, 251-3
    high frequency, 258-9
    infra-red radiation, 254-5
    radiant heat, 254-6
    safety precautions, 249-51
    sinusoidal currents, 253-4
    ultra-violet light, 256-8
Elevation, 117
Erector spinae, 163
Ethmoid bones, 109
Eversion, 116
Excretion, 184
Exercises, 182-231
    as aid to relaxation, 241-2
    at home, 201-2
    breathing, 235-40
    contra-indications, 186-7
    explanation by therapist, 203
    for mobility, 205-6, 222-7
    for obesity, 221-2
    for strengthening, 204-5, 228-33
    schemes, 192-6
    starting positions, 194, 195-6, 203
Expiration, 235
Extensor muscles, 46, 144-5, 154-6,
    158
External oblique, 167
Eyes, 83-4, 109

Face
    massage, 7, 27, 83-4
    muscles, 169-70
    position of lymph glands, 21
Faradism, 253-4
Fascia, 136-7
Fatty pads in joints, 115
Fatty tissue, 39
    effect of clapping, 33
    effect of massage, 48-9

Fatty tissue—*continued*
  effect of skin rolling, 30
  effect of wringing, 29
  treated by hacking, 32
Feet, 93
  bones, 103–5
  exercises, 227–8, 233
  finger kneading, 27–8
  flat, 263
  joints, 126–7
  massage technique, 68
  muscles, 157–8
  passive movements, 178–9
  remedying stiffness, 86
Femoral triangle, 21, 66, 75, 151
Femur, 100–1
Fibrositis, 31, 261
Fibula, 102–3
Fingers, 98
  joints, 123
  massage technique, 64–5
  passive movements, 176–7
  remedying stiffness, 86
Finland, 3
Flat back, 213
Flat feet, 263
Flexion, 115–16
Flexor muscles, 46, 142–3, 156–7
Floors, 16
Follicles, 24
Foramen magnum, 110
Forehead, 108
France, 5
French chalk, 41
Frictions, 6, 19, 25, 30–1, 61–2, 64, 67, 69, 71–2
  effects and uses, 31, 37, 45
Frontal bone, 108
Frozen shoulder, 262

Galen, 4
Galvanic current, 251–3
Gastrocnemius, 155

Girdles, 91–2
Glandular obesity, 40
Gluteal mass, 28, 29, 66, 72
Gluteal muscles, 147, 148
Gout, 50
Gracilis, 152
Gravity, 189–90, 194
Groin, *see* Femoral triangle
Gyratory, 274

Hacking, 19, 29, 31–3, 43, 49–50, 63–9, 71–2, 76, 79, 83
Haemophilia, 40
Hair, 12
  growth, 24
  superfluous, 267
Hairy areas, 22, 40, 41
Hand creams, 5–6
Hands, 13, 93
  bones, 97–8
  care, 43
  exercises, 42
  massage, 27–8, 64–5
  muscles, 146–7
  passive movements, 176
  remedying stiffness, 86
Hanging position, 196, 198–9
Head
  exercises, 228–9
  massage, 49, 82
  passive movements, 180–1
Heart, 45, 46
Heat production, 29, 32, 44
Heat treatments, 87
Heel bone, *see* Calcaneum
Hera, 2
Hernia, 40
High frequency electrical treatment, 258–9
Hip bones, 91, 99
Hip joints, 93, 99, 125
  exercises, 226–7, 231–2
  passive movements, 177–8, 179

Hip joints—*continued*
  remedying stiffness, 86
Humerus, 61, 95, 96
Hyperanaemia, 27, 31
Hyoid bone, 110

Iliac crests, 69, 70, 74, 75, 78
Iliac fossa, 78
Iliacus, 151
Iliad, 2
Ilium, 99, 100
Impetigo, 266
Incorporated Society of Trained
  Masseuses, 7
Infra-red radiation, 254–5
Infra-spinatus muscles, 69, 138
Injuries, 39
Insomnia, 23
Inspiration, 235
Institute of Massage and Remedial
  Exercise (Manchester), 7
Insulation, 249
Intercarpal joints, 122–3
Intercostal muscles, 108
Intermetacarpal joints, 123
Intermetatarsal joints, 127
Interossei, 157
Interphalangeal joints, 124, 127
Intertarsal joints, 126–7
Inversion, 116
Involuntary muscles, 24
Ironing, 70, 72
Ischium, 99, 100

Jaw, 129
Jaw bone, *see* Mandible
Jewellery, 12
Joints, 88, 111–30, 173
  classification, 111–13
  effect of massage, 28, 31, 45–6, 85–7
  movement, 115, 18, 130, 188–9
  types, 111–14

Kitchens, 16
Kneading, 5, 19, 24–8, 45, 60–73,
  76–8, 82–3
Knee bone, *see* Patella
Knee joints, 93, 125
  massage, 67, 86, 178–9
Kneeling position, 196, 198, 200
Kypho-Lordosis, 212–13
  See also Lordosis
Kyphosis, 211–12

Lacrymal bones, 109
Latissimus dorsi, 158, 159, 160
Legs, 93
  bones, 98–105
  exercises, 227–8, 233
  joints, 124–7
  massage programme, 57–8, 65–8
  muscles, 150, 154–6
  passive movements, 177–9
  position of lymph glands, 21
Lethargy, 24
Levator anguli oris, 170
Levator labii, 170
Levator palpebrae superioris, 170
Levator scapuli, 161
Levers, 187–8, 194
Ligaments, 113–14
Lighting, 53
Linen, 15, 52
Ling, Peter Henry, 6
Liver, 34, 36, 50
  massage, 76
Loofahs, 3
Lordosis, 210–11
  See also Kypho-Lordosis
Lubricants, 15
Lumbago, 262
Lumbricals, 157
Lungs, 33, 36, 47, 234
Lying position, 196–7, 200
Lymph, 36, 81
  flow, 21

Lymph glands, 20, 21, 46

Mandible, 110
Manipulations, 5
  effects summarized, 36
  groups, 19
  percussion, 31–5
  pressure, 24–31
  shaking, 35–6
  strength, 43
  stroking, 20–4
  technique, 20
Manubrium, 107
Massage
  contra-indications, 39–40
  definition, 1, 19
  effects summarized, 36
  full body, 56–9
  general method, 55–6
  history, 1–8
  psychological effects, 38–9, 44–51
  technique, 42–3
  use in physiotherapy, 7
Maxillae, 109
Medical histories, 17
Medical staff, 12–13, 17
Mentalis, 170
Metabolism, 50–1
Metacarpo-phalangeal joints, 124
Metacarpus, 98
Metatarso-phalangeal joints, 127
Metatarsus, 104
Midcarpal joints, 122–3
Mobility exercises, 205–6
Mouth, 84
Movement
  axes, 188–9
  mechanics, 187–91
  planes, 188, 189
  range, 190–1
Mucus, 33
Muscles, 114, 131–70
  action on joints, 134–6

Muscles—*continued*
  attachment, 132
  blood supply, 136
  building by exercise, 202–3
  contraction, 80, 133–4
  effect of beating and pounding, 34
  effect of circular kneading, 26, 27
  effect of exercises, 182–3
  effect of hacking, 32
  effect of massage, 44–5
  effect of wringing, 29
  flabby, 80
  increasing resistance, 195
  insertion, 89, 132
  origins, 89, 132
  range of movement, 190–1
  relaxation, 243
  shape, 132–3
  slack, 85
  structure, 132
  tissue types, 131
  tone, 134, 173–4
  types of work, 191
Music, 16, 192

Naevus, 267
Navel, 76, 77
Navicular bone, 103, 104
Neck
  exercises, 223–4, 228–9
  massage, 29, 49, 57, 58, 72
  muscles, 163, 165
  passive movements, 180–1
Nerve endings, 21, 48
Nervous system, 24, 32
  effect of exercise, 185
  effect of massage, 49
  in joints, 115
  in muscles, 136
Neuralgia, 4, 40
Neuritis, 40
Noise, 53
Nose bones, 109

Obesity, 24, 40, 50, 219–33
   treatment, 79, 221–2
   types, 220
   See also Slimming
Obturator foramen, 100
Occipital bone, 109, 110
Occipito frontalis, 170
Odyssey, 2
Oedema, 81–2
   See also Swellings
Oils, 1, 6, 41
Olecranon fossa, 96
Olecranon process, 96
Olive oil, 41
Orbicularis oculi, 170
Orbicularis oris, 170
Os innominatum, *see* Hip bones
Osteo-arthritis, 260

Pain relief, 87
Palmaris longus, 142
Passive movements, 171–81
   as substitute for exercise, 174–5
   contra-indications, 172
   effects and uses, 172–5
   techniques, 175–81
Patella, 67, 86, 103
Pectineus, 151
Pectoral muscles, 45, 60, 73, 163,
   165–6
Pelvic girlde, 92
Pelvic tilt, 209–10
Percussion, 19, 31–5, 37
   See also Beating; Clapping; Hack-
   ing; Pounding
Perfumes, 1, 6
Periosteum, 27, 45, 88
Peristalsis, 25, 34, 49, 184
Peroneus brevis, 155
Peroneus longus, 155
Peroneus tertius, 154
Petrissage, 6, 24, 25, 28
Phalanges, 98, 104–5

Phlebitis, 39
Physiotherapy, 7
Picking up, 19, 24, 28–9, 37, 61–7,
   69–70, 72, 78
Pillows, 14, 20
Pinching, 6
Pisiform, 98
Plantaris, 156
Platysma, 163, 165, 170
Point hacking, *see* Hacking
Popliteus, 156
Position of client and therapist, 6,
   14–15
   for abdominal massage, 74
   for face massage, 83
   for head and scalp massage, 82
   for lower back, 69–70
   for neck and chest massage, 72
   for upper back massage, 68–9
Posture, 46, 193, 201–2, 206–9
   effect of poor muscle tone, 44–5
   inspection for defects, 206–8
   specific conditions, 209–19
   static corrections, 208
   See also Spine
Pounding, 19, 34–5, 43, 72
Powder, 6, 15, 41
Pregnancy, 40
Pressure manipulations, 5, 6, 19,
   24–31, 45
   depth, 14
   effects and uses, 37
   See also Frictions; Ironing; Knead-
   ing; Picking up; Skin rolling;
   Wringing
Procerus, 170
Pronatur quadratus, 143
Pronatur teres, 142
Psoriasis, 265
Psoas, 151
Psychological effects, 38–9, 44–51
Pubic-symphesis joint, 124–5
Pubis, 99, 100

Punctuality, 11

Quadratus lumborum, 168
Quadriceps, 66

Radial fossa, 96
Radiant heat, 254–6
Radio-ulnar joints, 121
Radius, 96–7
Rate of movement, 13
Reception of clients, 16, 53
Record cards, 17, 52, 53
Rectus abdominis, 167
Rectus femoris, 66, 149
Red Cross, 38
Relaxation, 20, 26–7, 54, 240–7
    aided by beauty salons, 38
    as a philosophy, 241
    by heat treatments, 87
    effect of vibrations, 35
    mental, 244
    modification of treatment, 79–80,
        84–5
    of muscles, 243
    of therapist, 55
    starting position, 243
    technique, 245–7
    through passive movements, 172–3
Respiration, *see* Breathing
Rheumatism, 3, 40
Rheumatoid arthritis, 260
Rhomboid major, 162
Rhomboid minor, 162
Rhythm, 6, 13, 43
Ribs, 74, 107–8, 128
Risorius, 170
Romans, 2–3, 4
Rotation, 117

Sacro-iliac joint, 128–9
Sacrum, 34, 40, 91, 106
Safety precautions, 249–51
Sartorius, 151

Scalp, 24
    massage, 82
    muscles, 169
Scaphoid, 98
Scapula, 26, 69, 91, 94, 214–15
Scar tissue, 22, 31, 35, 40, 53, 74, 87
Sciatica, 262–3
Scoliosis, 214
Screens, 15
Scrubbing brushes, 3
Sebaceous glands, 21
Sebum, 21, 24
Secretions, 184
Semimembranosus, 153
Semitendinosus, 153
Sensitivity, 42
Serratus anterior, 163, 166
Serratus posterior superior, 163
Shaking, 20, 35–6, 38, 49–50
    See also Vibrations
Sheets, 15
Shin, 102
Shoes, 12
Shoulder girdle, 27, 60, 91
Shoulder joints, 93, 119–20
    passive movements, 175, 180
    remedying stiffness, 85
Shoulders, 26
    exercises, 222–4, 228–9
    frozen, 262
    massage, 49, 60–1
    muscles, 138–9
Sinusoidal currents, 253–4
Sitting position, 196, 197, 200
Skeleton, 88
Skin, 25
    capillaries, 23
    defects, 264–7
    dirty, 41
    diseases, 40
    effect of massage, 21, 47–8
    effect of oils, 41
    slack, 85

Skin rolling, 6, 19, 24, 25, 30, 37, 71, 79
Skull, 108–10
  joints, 129
Slapping, 6
Slimming
  aided by heat treatments, 87
  aided by massage, 48–9
  benefits of abdominal massage, 73
  in Middle Ages, 5
  See also Obesity
Slipped disk, 263
Small intestine, 76
Soap, 41
Society of Trained Masseuses, 7
Soleus, 156
Solicitors, 17
Spa towns, 4
Speed, 43
Sphenoid bones, 109
Spine, 31
  inspection for posture defects, 206–8
  passive movements, 179–80
  remedying stiffness, 86
  See also Posture; Vertebral column
Splenius capitus, 163
Splenius cervicus, 163
Staff rooms, 16
Stamina, 11
Stance, 14
  See also Position of client and therapist
Standing position, 196–9
Steam treatments, 87
Sterno-clavicular joint, 119
Sterno-mastoid muscle, 73, 85, 163, 165
Sternum, 91, 107
Stimulation, 80
Strengthening exercises, 204–5
Stroking, 19, 20–4, 37, 75–8, 82–3
  See also Effleurage
Styloid process, 96

Sub-cutaneous tissues, 25, 30, 34
Subscapularis, 139
Sudiferous glands, 47
Superfluous hairs, 267
Supinator, 145
Supra-clavicular glands, 21, 60, 69, 70
Supra-spinatus muscles, 69, 138
Surgical spirit, 41, 43
Sweat glands, *see* Sudiferous glands
Sweden, 6
Swellings, 22, 23, 40, 81
  See also Oedema
Switzerland, 5
Symphesis pubis, 91
Synovial membrane, 113
  See also Joints: synovial

Talus, 103
Tapotement, *see* Percussion manipulations
Tapping, *see* Hacking
Tarsal joint, 127
Tarsus, 103–4
Tax, 17
Teeth, 12
Temperature, 40
Temple, 109
Temporal bones, 109
Temporo-mandibular joint, 129
Tendons, 136
Tennis elbow, 261–2
Tenosynovitis, 261
Tension, 54, 173
  headaches, 23
Tensor fasciae femoris, 148
Teres major, 139
Teres minor, 139
Thigh bone, *see* Femur
Thighs, 93
  exercises, 226–7, 231–2
  muscles, 147, 149, 151, 152–3
Thoracic organs, 36
Thoracic vertebrae, 69, 105, 106

Thorax, 47, 107
Thrombosis, 39
Thumbs, 123
Tibia, 102, 103
Tibial muscles, 67, 154, 156
Toes
  bones, 104–5
  joints, 86, 127
Toilets, 16
Towels, 3, 15, 41
Trachea, 234
Transversalis, 168
Trapezius, 60, 69, 73, 85, 98, 158–9,
  160
Triceps, 61, 62, 140
Trolleys, 15
Tuberculosis, 33
Tumours, 39

Ulna, 96
Ultra-violet light, 256–8
Uniforms, 11

Varicose veins, 22, 39, 53
Vastus intermedus, 149
Vastus lateralis, 149

Vastus medialis, 149
Venous circulation, 20, 25, 46
Ventilation, 16
Vertebrae, 60, 105–6
Vertebral column, 105
  curves, 106–7
  joints, 128–9
  slipped disk, 263
  See also Spine
Vibrations, 6, 20, 35, 38, 50, 73, 77–8,
  82–3
Visceroptosis, 215, 216

Waist exercises, 224–5, 226, 230–1
Warmth, 14, 16
Warts, 267
Wash basins, 16
Wax treatments, 87
Weight lifting, 202–3
Winged scapula, 214–15
Wounds, 40
Wringing, 19, 24, 25, 29, 61–2, 64–6,
  69, 70, 72, 78
Wrist joints, 64, 86, 93, 122, 176

Zygomatic bones, 109, 170